Stanley Paul, PhD, OTR/L
Cindee Q. Peterson, PhD, O
Editors

Interprofessional Collaboration in Occupational Therapy

Interprofessional Collaboration in Occupational Therapy has been co-published simultaneously as *Occupational Therapy in Health Care*, Volume 15, Numbers 3/4 2001.

Pre-publication
REVIEWS,
COMMENTARIES,
EVALUATIONS . . .

"A GOOD SOURCE OF INFORMATION . . . . Introduces the reader to the concept of interprofessional collaboration, its benefits, barriers, and strategies for developing such collaboration . . . . Presents a series of research studies that show the value of interprofessional collaboration to achieve outcomes at different levels and within different service delivery models."

Dyhalma Irizarry, PhD, OTR/L, FAOTA
Director, Occupational Therapy Program, University of Puerto Rico

Interprofessional Collaboration in Occupational Therapy

Interprofessional Collaboration in Occupational Therapy has been co-published simultaneously as *Occupational Therapy in Health Care*, Volume 15, Numbers 3/4 2001.

The *Occupational Therapy in Health Care* Monographic "Separates"

Below is a list of "separates," which in serials librarianship means a special issue simultaneously published as a special journal issue or double-issue *and* as a "separate" hardbound monograph. (This is a format which we also call a "DocuSerial.")

"Separates" are published because specialized libraries or professionals may wish to purchase a specific thematic issue by itself in a format which can be separately cataloged and shelved, as opposed to purchasing the journal on an on-going basis. Faculty members may also more easily consider a "separate" for classroom adoption.

"Separates" are carefully classified separately with the major book jobbers so that the journal tie-in can be noted on new book order slips to avoid duplicate purchasing.

You may wish to visit Haworth's website at . . .

http://www.HaworthPress.com

. . . to search our online catalog for complete tables of contents of these separates and related publications.

You may also call 1-800-HAWORTH (outside US/Canada: 607-722-5857), or Fax: 1-800-895-0582 (outside US/Canada: 607-771-0012), or e-mail at:

getinfo@haworthpressinc.com

Interprofessional Collaboration in Occupational Therapy, edited by Stanley Paul, PhD, OTR/L, and Cindee Q. Peterson, PhD, OTR (Vol. 15, No. 3/4, 2001). *"A GOOD SOURCE OF INFORMATION. . . . Introduces the reader to the concept of interprofessional collaboration, its benefits, barriers, and strategies for developing such collaboration. . . . Presents a series of research studies that show the value of interprofessional collaboration to achieve outcomes at different levels and within different service delivery models." (Dyhalma Irizarry, PhD, OTR/L, FAOTA, Director, Occupational Therapy Program, University of Puerto Rico)*

Education for Occupational Therapy in Health Care: Strategies for the New Millennium, edited by Patricia Grist, PhD, OTR/L, FAOTA, and Marjorie Scaffa, PhD, OTR/L, FAOTA (Vol. 15, No. 1/2, 2001). *"PROVIDES TRULY IMAGINATIVE IDEAS for preparing the practitioners of the near future–and not a moment too soon! It is easy to see that these authors have been outstanding clinicians. . . . they put their OT skills to work in creating these unique learning-by-doing educational packages. Especially exciting are the clever ways in which alternative sites and programs are used to provide fieldwork experiences." (Nedra P. Gillette, MEd, OTR, ScD (Hon), Director, Institute for the Study of Occupation and Health, American Occupational Therapy Foundation)*

Community for Occupational Therapy Education and Practice, edited by Beth P. Velde, PhD, OTR/L, and Peggy Prince Wittman, EdD, OTR/L, FAOTA (Vol. 13, No. 3/4, 2001). *"Introduces the concept of commuity-based practice in non-traditional settings. Whether one is concerned with wellness and the aging process or with debilitating situations, injuries, or diseases such as homelessness, AIDS, or multiple sclerosis, this collection details the process of moving forward." (Scott D. McPhee, DrPH, OT, FAOTA, Associate Dean and Chair, School of Occupational Therapy, Belmont University, Nashville, Tennessee)*

Interprofessional Collaboration in Occupational Therapy

Stanley Paul, PhD, OTR/L
Cindee Q. Peterson, PhD, OTR
Editors

Interprofessional Collaboration in Occupational Therapy has been co-published simultaneously as *Occupational Therapy in Health Care*, Volume 15, Numbers 3/4 2001.

The Haworth Press, Inc.
New York • London • Oxford

Interprofessional Collaboration in Occupational Therapy has been co-published simultaneously as *Occupational Therapy in Health Care*™, Volume 15, Numbers 3/4 2001.

Cover design by Thomas J. Mayshock, Jr.

Library of Congress Cataloging-in-Publication Data

Interprofessional collaboration in occupational therapy/Stanley Paul, Cindee Q. Peterson, editors.
    p.; cm.
"Co-published simultaneously as: Occupational therapy in health care, volume 15, numbers 3/4 2001."
Includes bibliographical references.
    ISBN 0-7890-1902-7 (hard: alk. paper) --ISBN 0-7890-1903-5 (pbk: alk. paper)
1. Health care teams. 2. Occupational therapy--Practice.
    [DNLM: 1. Occupational Therapy--methods. 2. Interprofessional Relations. 3. Physical Therapy Techniques--methods. WB 555 I61 2002]
I. Paul, Stanley, 1964- II. Peterson, Cindee Quake, 1953- III. Occupational therapy in health care.
RM735.4. I584 2002
615.8'515--dc21   2002002899

Indexing, Abstracting & Website/Internet Coverage

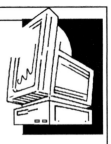

This section provides you with a list of major indexing & abstracting services. That is to say, each service began covering this periodical during the year noted in the right column. Most Websites which are listed below have indicated that they will either post, disseminate, compile, archive, cite or alert their own Website users with research-based content from this work. (This list is as current as the copyright date of this publication.)

(continued)

Special Bibliographic Notes related to special journal issues (separates) and indexing/abstracting:

- indexing/abstracting services in this list will also cover material in any "separate" that is co-published simultaneously with Haworth's special thematic journal issue or DocuSerial. Indexing/abstracting usually covers material at the article/chapter level.
- monographic co-editions are intended for either non-subscribers or libraries which intend to purchase a second copy for their circulating collections.
- monographic co-editions are reported to all jobbers/wholesalers/approval plans. The source journal is listed as the "series" to assist the prevention of duplicate purchasing in the same manner utilized for books-in-series.
- to facilitate user/access services all indexing/abstracting services are encouraged to utilize the co-indexing entry note indicated at the bottom of the first page of each article/chapter/contribution.
- this is intended to assist a library user of any reference tool (whether print, electronic, online, or CD-ROM) to locate the monographic version if the library has purchased this version but not a subscription to the source journal.
- individual articles/chapters in any Haworth publication are also available through the Haworth Document Delivery Service (HDDS).

Interprofessional Collaboration in Occupational Therapy

CONTENTS

ABOUT THE EDITORS

Stanley Paul, PhD, OTR/L, is Associate Professor in the Department of Occupational Therapy at Western Michigan University. He completed his doctoral degree at New York University and his post-professional master's degree at the University of Buffalo. He has practiced as an OT clinician in the areas of physical disabilities, pediatrics, and developmental disabilities. His research interests include outcome studies of occupational therapy services, assistive technology and functional independence of individuals with disabilities, adaptive design and productivity, students with disabilities in higher education, and aging and function. He is presently engaged in a grant-funded multi-stage research project that examines the role of various physical environmental factors on mobility and function in community-dwelling elderly. Dr. Paul has a number of research publications in various occupational therapy, allied health, and medical journals.

Cindee Q. Peterson, PhD, OTR, is Professor and Chair, Department of Occupational Therapy at Western Michigan University. She completed her doctoral degree at The Union Institute in Cincinnati and her master's degree in counseling psychology at Western Michigan University. She has practiced as an OT clinician in the areas of pediatrics, developmental disabilities, and mental illness. Her research interests include attention deficit disorder, handwriting, and purposeful occupation. Dr. Peterson currently serves on the National Advisory Committee on Interdisciplinary, Community Based Linkages as part of the Health Resources and Services Administration (HRSA). She was appointed to the Committee by the former United States Secretary of Health and Human Services, Donna Shalala.

Interprofessional Collaboration: Issues for Practice and Research

Stanley Paul, PhD, OTR/L
Cindee Q. Peterson, PhD, OTR

SUMMARY. The current health care system is based on accountability, cost containment, and quality of care. Collaborative practice models may be a viable means for improving health care delivery. The purpose of this paper is to outline how interprofessional education, practice, and research can establish economic benefits and effective clinical outcomes outside of discipline specific investigation. *[Article copies available for a fee from The Haworth Document Delivery Service: 1-800-HAWORTH. E-mail address: <getinfo@haworthpressinc.com> Website: <http://www.HaworthPress.com> © 2001 by The Haworth Press, Inc. All rights reserved.]*

KEYWORDS. Practice models, health care delivery

Stanley Paul is Associate Professor, Department of Occupational Therapy, College of Health and Human Services, Western Michigan University, Kalamazoo, MI 49008 (E-mail: stanley.paul@wmich.edu).

Cindee Q. Peterson is Professor and Chair, Department of Occupational Therapy, College of Health and Human Services, Western Michigan University, Kalamazoo, MI 49008 (E-mail: cindee.peterson@wmich.edu). Cindee Peterson is currently a member of the National Advisory Committee on Interdisciplinary Community-Based Linkages appointed by the Secretary of Health and Human Services, Washington, DC.

[Haworth co-indexing entry note]: "Interprofessional Collaboration: Issues for Practice and Research." Paul, Stanley, and Cindee Q. Peterson. Co-published simultaneously in *Occupational Therapy in Health Care* (The Haworth Press, Inc.) Vol. 15, No. 3/4, 2001, pp. 1-12; and: *Interprofessional Collaboration in Occupational Therapy* (ed: Stanley Paul, and Cindee Q. Peterson) The Haworth Press, Inc., 2001, pp. 1-12. Single or multiple copies of this article are available for a fee from The Haworth Document Delivery Service [1-800-HAWORTH, 9:00 a.m. - 5:00 p.m. (EST). E-mail address: getinfo@haworthpressinc.com].

1

Traditional health care delivery has focused on acute illnesses and symptom correction that lead to service delivery through a multidisciplinary model. Several factors have resulted in an urgent need to improve the health care delivery system in the 21st century. A changing population of elderly, uninsured, and individuals with complex chronic illnesses due to increased survival rates, has increased the need for health care professionals in a time of limited resources (Simpson et al., 2001). Managed care organizations have not been able to offer consistent quality of care resulting in dissatisfaction of the public and professionals within the current delivery systems.

Collaborative practice models may address the needs of the elderly, underserved, and chronically ill more effectively than traditional primary care models that are experiencing shortages of health care professionals. The federal government, across numerous funding agencies, has established funding priorities aimed at quality of care and life-significant outcomes across disciplines. In order to address the health care needs of the nation, a national acceptance of interdisciplinary health care must occur. No discipline possesses all the skills and knowledge needed to address factors of improved health and health care within complex systems designed to meet those needs (Headrick, 2001). Interprofessional education and practice can only be established through research to determine economic benefits and effective clinical outcomes. An interprofessional team conducting research provides an innovative approach that cannot be achieved by discipline specific investigators (Laskin et al., 2001). Evidence of the value of interdisciplinary health care is needed to determine patient or provider satisfaction and cost-benefit, cost-effectiveness, or cost-neutral impact.

WHAT IS INTERPROFESSIONAL COLLABORATION?

Interprofessional collaboration is a newer term used in current literature for interdisciplinary collaboration involving health professions (Baldwin, 1996). The term interdisciplinary is considered confusing because subspecialists within professional disciplines may consider collaborative work interdisciplinary (Simpson et al., 2001). Interprofessional collaboration in health care is a partnership among different professionals for the purpose of providing quality health care to individuals and communities (Simpson et al., 2001). Collaboration occurs when a group of individuals with diverse backgrounds work together as a unit to solve patient problems, set up mutual goals, work interdependently to define and treat patient problems, accept and capitalize on disciplinary differences, share leadership, and communicate effectively with each other (Perkins & Tryssenaar, 1994).

THREE MODELS OF PROFESSIONAL COLLABORATION

In a multidisciplinary model each health professional does his or her work separately. Even though members share their findings with other team members, each team member provides the services described in his/her assessment and plan separately (Angelo, 1997). Hierarchical authority often exists in a multidisciplinary model (Greenberg & Bellack, 1999); each profession behaves with different perspectives and relationships are limited and transitory (Angelo, 1997).

In an interprofessional model, clients may be assessed separately or with other professionals. An integrated plan is formulated, but each professional retains the responsibility of providing the services he or she recommended (Angelo, 1997). Here, the individuals with varied disciplinary training coordinate their activities to provide services to a client (Perkins & Tryssenaar, 1994). Unlike a multidisciplinary model, members of an interprofessional health care team interact with each other before and after their individual interventions with the patient. On some occasions they may co-treat a patient while working on a number of goals concurrently.

In a transdisciplinary model, professional lines blur more often than the other two models. Assessments, treatment plans, and interventions are often carried out jointly. Role exchange may occur during the intervention stage where a different professional might carry out a program recommended by another professional. Severe role blurring is seen as a serious disadvantage of a transdisciplinary model (Clay et al., 1999).

Even though each of these models has its strengths and weaknesses, interprofessional models have gained popularity due to changing health care needs and the shortcomings of the traditional multidisciplinary model (Clay et al., 1999). In a traditional health care model there is a hierarchy starting with the physician followed by other professionals. In an interprofessional model each professional is respected as a team member rather than as a subordinate and each contributes equally to the welfare of the patient.

INTERPROFESSIONAL COLLABORATION IN CLINICAL PRACTICE

According to Simpson et al. (2001), there is a need for evidence-based models for the conduct and coordination of care in all health care settings. The literature suggests a lack of published studies on interprofessional practice involving occupational therapy. An interdisciplinary in-service training program at the University of Chicago designed to improve early childhood occupational therapy and physical therapy services was one of few models cited (Lawlor & Cada, 1994). A number of factors were identified as prohibitive to the development of successful interdisciplinary models. These factors included an unclear definition of interprofessional practice, a lack of data on cost-effectiveness, and a lack of theoretical and conceptual clarity about interprofessional collaboration (Simpson et al., 2001).

Interprofessional collaboration can be an effective disability management model and an effective framework for prevention and intervention. Several articles in this volume on interdisciplinary practice outline successful interprofessional service delivery models inclusive of occupational therapy. The Rural Elderly Assessment Project (REAP), a Health Resources and Services Administration (HRSA) sponsored project, demonstrates a collaborative effort to train occupational therapy, physical therapy, physician assistant, and public health students to conduct interdisciplinary team health assessments with rural, community-dwelling older adults (Miller & Ishler, 2001). The Child Trauma Assessment Center (CTAC) describes a collaborative partnership in the delivery of services to children who have been traumatized by abuse, neglect, and prenatal exposure to alcohol (Hyter et al., 2001). Members of the CTAC team include the disciplines of counseling, occupational therapy, pediatric medicine, social work, and speech-language pathology. The Microwave Project for community elders is an example of a collaborative relationship between occupational therapy and a community agency involved in providing meals for elderly people who are homebound (Miller et al., in press).

BENEFITS OF INTERPROFESSIONAL COLLABORATION

Some of the benefits of interprofessional collaboration include:

• Opportunities for professionals to work collaboratively on patient goals

- Professional competence in working independently as well as in interprofessional teams
- Evidence-based decision making, shared responsibility, and public accountability
- Cost-effective use of resources, opportunities to make referrals to other professions, and avoiding duplication of services
- Effective use of faculty time and physical space by teaching subjects that are common to different health professions, e.g., anatomy, physiology, kinesiology, and other basic sciences.
- Interaction between students of different professions leads to respect, cooperation and knowledge about other professions rather than envy or disrespect.
- There is increasing proof on the effectiveness of interprofessional education. Research has shown improved student performance, client/family satisfaction, and changes in attitudes among different professionals in interprofessional educational settings (Baldwin, 1994; Curley et al., 1998; Wartmann et al., 1998).
- Academic Health Education Centers that employ interprofessional training find the practice to be efficient and cost-effective in today's marketplace.

BARRIERS TO INTERPROFESSIONAL COLLABORATION

Barriers to interprofessional collaboration include physical and attitudinal barriers. Some of these barriers include:

- Traditional educational separation and turf battle issues among disciplines. Attitudinal barriers that encourage isolationist policy that discourage collaboration with other professions
- Interprofessional teaching requires greater demands on faculty time due to the need for coordination with other professional members of the teaching team.
- Scheduling conflict for students to take interprofessional courses
- Curriculum content that follows a strict and narrow disciplinary line
- Physical barriers such as lack of clinical sites for interdisciplinary placement
- Differences in perceived value of collaboration among different professions

- Individual members' unique attitudes and styles of practice that is not conducive to teamwork
- Inadequate knowledge about different disciplines
- Value conflicts among different disciplines such as "saving life" (medical, illness-based concept) versus "quality of life and patient autonomy" paradigms
- A belief that interprofessional education is a fad and that traditional curricula will survive
- Current managed care demands to cut costs and show constant evidence about the discipline's unique effectiveness
- Need for funding for interprofessional research and training projects.

STRATEGIES FOR DEVELOPING INTERDISCIPLINARY COLLABORATION

A monolithic mode of professional education does not prepare a professional for the practical health care environment that requires multiple health professionals and a team approach. Adopting interprofessional education and practice requires change at the professional, personal, and institutional practice levels. Collaboration is a developmental process involving building relationships between different professions, as well as involving the client and family members into the decision-making process. Some strategies for developing interdisciplinary collaboration include:

- Profession's commitment to model effective interdisciplinary collaboration in teaching, research, and clinical practice (Clay et al., 1999).
- Develop interdisciplinary educational programs at college and university settings to promote working together with other disciplines.
- Incorporate planned interdisciplinary experiences in the curriculum through interdisciplinary seminars, courses, clinical experiences, some cross-training expectations, and collaborative research projects (Clay et al., 2001).
- Establish contacts with local rural and urban facilities that have interprofessional practice. For example, existing Academic Health Education Centers (AHEC) that provide opportunities for students of various disciplines to work together.

- Introduce interprofessional courses to AHECs, which do not have established interprofessional practice. A few interprofessional courses could include "introduction to rural health" and "communication skills for health professionals."
- Train and develop faculty and preceptors who are not familiar with interprofessional curriculum. Provide faculty rewards that acknowledge interprofessional work.
- Incorporate a service learning piece into collaborative education and practice in the community. For example, develop an interprofessional community-based model with a focus on service-learning for students and faculty.
- Community-based and campus-based programs for training students on interdisciplinary collaboration. For example, effective use of technology to link students from different professions on campus and during their service-based learning period in the community. Such community-based and campus-based interprofessional education can promote the value of innovation, teamwork, and accountability (Behringer et al., 1999).
- Educational exchange: According to Pew Health Professions Commission and the California Primary Care Consortium (1995), legitimate areas of specialized study should remain the domain of individual professional training, but key areas of clinical and preclinical training should be integrated across professional communities through sharing of training resources, more cross teaching, and more exploration of various roles played by different professionals.
- Identify barriers to interdisciplinary collaboration within the profession or department, discuss and analyze most significant barriers and develop strategies to overcome the barriers.
- Compile descriptions of different disciplines and their skills and knowledge important for collaborative practice.
- Seek funding sources to develop and continue interprofessional education and for interprofessional research and training projects.

INTERPROFESSIONAL COLLABORATION FOR OCCUPATIONAL THERAPY

Considering the constant need for interprofessional expertise, interprofessional collaboration in health care in the future may be inevitable. Interprofessional collaboration can be an effective disability management model. It can serve as an effective framework for prevention, rehabilitation, and maintenance of function. The following scenarios are a few examples of interprofessional collaboration:

- Physical therapy and occupational therapy working on a functional goal
- Speech pathology and occupational therapy working on a communication goal
- Nursing and occupational therapy working on a positioning goal
- Social work and occupational therapy working on a return to work/school goal
- Engineering and occupational therapy working on an assistive technology goal, and
- Collaboration between occupational therapy and neurology in the management of spasticity of the hand by identifying the most functional position for a neuronal block.

Other specialized areas where collaboration may be needed include:

- An occupational therapy case manager of an adult day care program requiring knowledge about the different disciplines involved in the program
- Interdisciplinary collaboration with physical therapy and speech pathology in an early intervention program, and
- A structured academic experience for medical, nursing, occupational therapy, and physical therapy students in an interprofessional care of geriatric clients.

INTERPROFESSIONAL ACTIVITIES FOR OCCUPATIONAL THERAPY

Occupational therapy should identify specific interprofessional objectives, devise a plan to meet those objectives, and develop specific activities and methods for carrying out the plan. Some specific activities include:

- Identifying effective models for occupational therapy to collaborate with different disciplines
- Interprofessional home visits
- Interprofessional case conferences

- Interprofessional community-based clinical experiences
- Presentations and publications with interprofessional colleagues, and
- Collaborative research that will help validate the profession.

DOES INTERPROFESSIONAL COLLABORATION WORK?

The advantages of interprofessional collaboration in health care are well-documented in the literature; it can be an effective tool to solving the various issues faced in today's health care. Studies have shown the effectiveness of interprofessional collaboration with successful patient outcomes, reduction in health care costs, patient satisfaction, worker satisfaction, and enhancement of professional identity within the health care system (Lewis, 1999; Murdaugh et al., 1999; Rice, 2000). Koppel and colleagues (2001) carefully reviewed the effectiveness involving interprofessional education in 10 health professions. Out of the 99 cases studied, only a handful of cases showed neutral or negative outcomes. Future research should compare different models of practice to further validate the effectiveness of interprofessional collaboration.

CONCLUSION

Today's health care system is based on accountability, cost containment, and quality of care. The shift in focus has been outcome and highest quality of service for the least cost. Comprehensive, evidence-based interprofessional models are very appropriate for effective practice. Evidence comparing patient outcome, patient and family satisfaction, and cost effectiveness of the traditional and interprofessional models of practice is needed (Clay et al., 2001).

Evidence-based health care is not limited to the United States but is becoming prevalent in other countries. The World Health Organization (WHO) has advocated the usefulness of interprofessional teamwork (WHO, 1988). Patient care is delivered by teams, not by individuals. Complex conditions require joint care by various health providers. Thus teamwork is not optional but mandatory. For example, one specific profession cannot meet all the needs of patients. A neurologist cannot meet the occupational therapy goals of a patient and a physiatrist may not be able to meet the psychosocial needs of a patient.

The continuing changes in health care appear to support a shift toward teamwork, collaboration, and reintegration of knowledge instead of the period dominated by individual professional experts and specialists. This calls for development of an interprofessional culture, building successful interprofessional experiences for students, faculty, and researchers. As the Pew report points out, in the future of health care provision, all health professionals including physicians, nurses, allied health professions, and public health officials need to work together (O'Neil & the Pew Health Professions Commission, 1998). Thus, in the long run, a multidisciplinary model to practice may not prove to be cost effective.

Interprofessional collaboration presents opportunities for occupational therapy to advance knowledge and skills for effective practice. The advantages of collaborative practice have been identified in the early occupational therapy literature (Weiss, 1977). The benefits of interprofessional collaboration appear to enrich educational experience, produce better health care professionals, and enhance patient care (Holmes & Osterweis, 1999). An interprofessional approach to occupational therapy practice will require a different mindset, skills, and educational training. As a final thought, is interprofessional collaboration the best way for the occupational therapy profession? Only continued evaluation and research will be able to answer the question.

REFERENCES

Angelo, J. (1997). *Assistive technology for rehabilitation therapists.* Philadelphia: F. A. Davis.

Baldwin, D. C. (1994). *The role of interdisciplinary education and teamwork in primary care and health reform.* Washington, DC: U. S. Department of Health and Human Services.

Baldwin, D. C. (1996). Some historical notes on interdisciplinary and interprofessional education and practice in health care in the USA. *Journal of Interprofessional Care, 10,* 173-187.

Behringer, B. A., Bishop, W. S., Edwards, J. B., & Franks, R. D. (1999). A model for partnerships among communities, disciplines, and institutions. In D. E. Holmes & M. Osterweis (Eds.), *Catalysts in interdisciplinary education* (pp. 43-58). Washington, DC: Association of Academic Health Centers.

Clay, M. C., Cummings, D. M., Greer, A. G., & Dreyfus, K. S. (2001). Developing interdisciplinary health sciences education: A collaborative university-community model. *Issues in Interdisciplinary Care, 3,* 69-75.

Clay, M. C., Cummings, D. M., Mansfield, C., & Hallock, J. A. (1999). Retooling to meet the needs of a changing health care system. In D. E. Holmes & M. Osterweis

(Eds.), *Catalysts in interdisciplinary education* (pp. 25-42). Washington, DC: Association of Academic Health Centers.

Curley, C., McEachern, J. E., & Speroff, T. (1998). A firm trial of interdisciplinary rounds on the inpatient medical wards: An intervention designed using continuous quality improvement. *Medical Care, 36,* AS 4-12.

Greenberg, R. S., & Bellack, J. P. (1999). Building an interdisciplinary culture. In D. E. Holmes & M. Osterweis (Eds.), *Catalysts in interdisciplinary education* (pp. 59-78). Washington, DC: Association of Academic Health Centers.

Headrick, L. A. (2001, January). *Interdisciplinary education in the service of others: Benefits and challenges.* Presentation to the National Advisory Committee on Interdisciplinary, Community-Based Linkages, Washington, DC.

Holmes, D. E., & Osterweis, M. (1999). What is past is prologue: Interdisciplinarity at the turn of the century. In D. E. Holmes & M. Osterweis (Eds.), *Catalysts in interdisciplinary education* (pp. 1-6). Washington, DC: Association of Academic Health Centers.

Hyter, Y. D., Atchison, B., Henry, J., Sloane, M., & Black-Pond, C. (2001). A response to traumatized children: Developing a best practices model. *Occupational Therapy in Health Care, 15* (3/4), 113-140.

Koppel, I., Barr, H., Reeves, S., Freeth, D., & Hammick, M. (2001). Establishing a systematic approach to evaluating the effectiveness of interprofessional education. *Issues in Interdisciplinary Care, 3,* 41-49.

Laskin, D. M., Augsberger, A., Hawkins, J., Olson, P., Rice, A., Soloway, M., & Ball, J. (2001). Interprofessional health care research: Recommendations of the National Academies of Practice Expert Panel on Health Care in the 21st Century. In J. A. Lewis (Ed.), *Issues in Interdisciplinary Care, 3,* 33-39.

Lawlor, M. C., & Cada, E. A. (1994). *The UIC Therapeutic Partnership Project. Final Report,* Chicago, IL: University of Illinois at Chicago.

Lewis, J. A. (1999). A new beginning. *National Academics of Practice Forum, 1,* 3.

Miller, B. K., & Ishler, K. J. (2001). The rural elderly assessment project: A model for interdisciplinary team training. *Occupational Therapy in Health Care, 15* (3/4), 13-34.

Miller, P. A., Hedden, J. L., Argento, L., Vaccaro, M., Murad, V., & Dionne, W. (In Press). A team approach to health promotion of community elders: The Microwave project. *Occupational Therapy in Health Care*

Murdaugh, C., Parsons, M., Gryb-Wysocki, T., Palmer, J., Glasby, C., Bonner, J., & Tavakoli, A. (1999). Implementing a quality of care model in a restructured hospital environment. *National Academics of Practice Forum, 1,* 219-226.

O'Neil, E. H., & Pew Health Professions Commission. (1988). *Recreating health professional practice for a new century.* San Francisco: Pew Health Professions Commission.

Perkins, J., & Tryssenaar, J. (1994). Making interdisciplinary education effective for rehabilitative students. *Journal of Allied Health, 23* (3), 133-141.

Rice, A. H. (2000). Interdisciplinary collaboration in health education, practice, and research. *National Academics of Practice Forum, 2* (1), 59-73.

Simpson, G., Rabin, D., Schmitt, M., Taylor, P., Urban, S., & Ball, J. W. (2001). Interprofessional health care practice: Recommendations of the National Academics of Practice Expert Panel on health care in the 21st century. *Issues in Interdisciplinary Care, 3,* 5-20.

Wartmann, S. A., Davis, A. K., Wilson, M. E. H., Kahn, N. B., & Kahn, R. H. (1998). Emerging lessons of the Interdisciplinary Generalist Curriculum (IGC) Project. *Academic Medicine, 73,* 935-942.

Weiss, M. W. (1977). Cooperative research in occupational therapy. *American Journal of Occupational Therapy, 31,* 44-45.

World Health Organization. (1988). *Learning together to work together for health.* (Tech. Rep. No. 769). Geneva, Switzerland: Author.

The Rural Elderly Assessment Project:
A Model for Interdisciplinary
Team Training

Barbara Kopp Miller, PhD
Karen J. Ishler, MA, LSW

SUMMARY. The Rural Elderly Assessment Project (REAP) was designed to train occupational therapy, physical therapy, physician assistant, and public health faculty and students to conduct interdisciplinary team health assessments with rural, community-dwelling older adults. This article highlights key features of the project's design and implementation and presents preliminary evaluation data from the 25 students who participated in the project. Students completed several pre- and post-test measures. Statistically significant improvements were observed in all but one of the knowledge, skill, and attitude domains that were specifically targeted by the project. Students identified a variety of benefits they received from participating in the project, and all students indicated that they would recommend the project to another student. Im-

Barbara Kopp Miller is Associate Professor, Department of Occupational Therapy, School of Allied Health, Medical College of Ohio, 3015 Arlington Ave., Rm. 4222, Toledo, OH 43614-5803 (E-mail: bkoppmiller@mco.edu).

Karen J. Ishler is Assistant Director, Western Reserve Geriatric Education Center, Case Western Reserve University in Cleveland, 12200 Fairhill Rd., Cleveland, OH 44120. Address correspondence to Dr. Kopp Miller.

[Haworth co-indexing entry note]: "The Rural Elderly Assessment Project: A Model for Interdisciplinary Team Training." Miller, Barbara Kopp, and Karen J. Ishler. Co-published simultaneously in *Occupational Therapy in Health Care* (The Haworth Press, Inc.) Vol. 15, No. 3/4, 2001, pp. 13-34; and: *Interprofessional Collaboration in Occupational Therapy* (ed: Stanley Paul, and Cindee Q. Peterson) The Haworth Press, Inc., 2001, pp. 13-34. Single or multiple copies of this article are available for a fee from The Haworth Document Delivery Service [1-800-HAWORTH, 9:00 a.m. - 5:00 p.m. (EST). E-mail address: getinfo@haworthpressinc.com].

13

plications for project replication and interdisciplinary team training of allied health students are discussed. *[Article copies available for a fee from The Haworth Document Delivery Service: 1-800-HAWORTH. E-mail address: <getinfo@haworthpressinc.com> Website: <http://www.HaworthPress.com> © 2001 by The Haworth Press, Inc. All rights reserved.]*

KEYWORDS. Geriatric, education, occupational therapy, gerontology, older adults

INTRODUCTION

The Rural Elderly Assessment Project (REAP) at the Medical College of Ohio was designed to prepare a group of allied health educators and students from occupational therapy, physical therapy, physician assistant and public health to work effectively as a health assessment team with rural, communty-dwelling, older adults. The goal of the REAP Project emerged from a synthesis of the literature on interdisciplinary team training and demographic statistics of rural, older adults. In addition, REAP was conceptualized from a broad base perspective. *A National Agenda for Geriatric Education: White Papers* (U. S. Department of Health and Human Services, 1996), *Healthy People 2000* (U. S. Department of Health and Human Services, 1990) and *Critical Challenges: Revitalizing the Health Professions for the Twenty-First Century* (Pew Health Professions Commission, 1995) provided the framework for the national and regional significance for REAP. A review of salient sources articulated the following three facts.

America's Population Is Aging and Living Longer with Chronic Conditions

Data from 1997 indicate that almost 13% of America's population is 65 years of age or older and will continue to grow significantly in the future (American Association of Retired Persons and Administration on Aging, 1998). Northwest Ohio, where REAP was conducted, reflects the national trend as indicated by the following statistics. Ohio statistics show that 13.4% of its population is over the age of 65 (Area Office on Aging of Northwest Ohio, Inc., 1994). Proportionally, northwest Ohio has one of the largest per capita population of elderly in the United States (Scripps Gerontology Center, 1990). The most significant area of growth will be the older age category 75 years of age and older where there will be a 13.5% increase in older adults (Northwest Ohio Health Planning, Inc., 1997). In addition, 55% of Ohio residents over the age of 65 live rurally without access to senior centers, malls, wellness clinics or other agencies that normally serve to promote health and quality of life.

The older adults that REAP served included those who lived in rural areas and/or medically underserved areas. The rural elderly living in medically underserved areas are becoming the oldest-old with multiple chronic illnesses which place them at risk for costly long-term or intermittent care (U. S. Department of Health and Human Services, 1996). As reported by Krout (1998), the majority of rural/urban comparison studies have provided evidence supporting the disadvantaged health status and great health and social service needs, of older rural adults. In addition, research suggests that chronic conditions are experienced at higher rates among the rural elderly placing them in greater need for accessible community-based services (Krout, 1994). In addition, evidence suggests that the elderly, both urban and rural, have increasing rates of related suicide, anxiety, alcohol and drug abuse (U. S. Department of Health and Human Services, 1996). Collectively, these factors speak to a need for great collaboration among health care professionals and agencies to identify and assess at-risk elderly and to intervene proactively in the creation of social, emotional, and environmental networks of prevention and support.

Managed Care Impacts Service Provision for the Elderly

The health care financing conundrum impacts the elderly more than any other age cohort. Fragmented financing, uncertain coverage, and fear prevent the elderly from seeking medical attention in a timely manner (U. S. Department of Health and Human Services, 1996). This results in a formerly manageable, chronic condition becoming a costly acute medical crisis. Medicare, Medicaid, the Older American Act funds, private health insurance, retiree benefits and out-of-pocket payments present a daunting health care management challenge for service care providers and recipients (U. S. Department of Health and Human Services, 1996). Medicare's rapid transition from a retrospective payment system to a prospective payment system has had a significant impact on service provision for the elderly. Shortened lengths of hospital and subacute care mean that the elderly will rely more on outpatient services, services in the home and rehabilitative care that focuses on timely assessment of risk, health promotion education and preventive education.

Cost barriers exist, however, that prevent the development and implementation of effective, interdisciplinary health promotion and prevention services (Mockenhaupt & Muchow, 1994).

Allied health professionals have important roles to play in health promotion and disease/dysfunction prevention. Allied health curricula need to go beyond providing academic theory related to health promotion and disease/dysfunction prevention and include practical experiences in providing programming within a context of an interdisciplinary team. The Pew Commission (O'Neil & Pew Health Professions Commission, 1998) has established a competency stating that all health care practitioners should rigorously practice preventive health care. They recommend that curricula teach principles of prevention, health promotion, risk reduction and behavior change. Further, they recommend that students be provided community-based learning experiences in health promotion and self-management of health with defined groups.

Health Care Professionals Need Education to Work Effectively in Interdisciplinary Teams if They Are to Meet the Needs of the Elderly

The Pew Health Professions Commission has identified 21 competencies for the twenty-first century for the next generation of health care professionals (O'Neil & Pew Health Professions Commission, 1998). The Commission has identified the ability to work in interdisciplinary teams as critical for assuring effective and efficient coordination of care. The Commission continues by writing that curricula should incorporate planned, interdisciplinary experiences and actively model effective interdisciplinary collaboration.

The literature suggests that interdisciplinary education and delivery of comprehensive health care services are desirable and beneficial. Some of the advantages associated with an interdisciplinary approach are increased efficiency and reduced costs, greater patient satisfaction, and a reduction in the use of medical services (Carstensen, Edelstein, & Dornbrand, 1996; U. S. Department of Health and Human Services, 1996). In the field of geriatrics, authors suggest that an interdisciplinary team approach to service delivery results in lower mortality, less frequent and shortened length of hospital stays, increased satisfaction on the part of consumers, reduced time spent in nursing homes, and improved functional status (Carstensen, Edelstein, & Dornbrand, 1996; U. S. Department of Health and Human Services, 1996). Finally, Pfeiffer (1999) argues that an interdisciplinary approach to caring for older adults is the only way health care professionals can meet the diverse needs of older adults.

Faculty and students have also reported benefits of participating in interdisciplinary curricula. For example, Buck, Tilson and Andersen (1999) reported that both students and faculty viewed the interdisciplinary experience as beneficial. Ninety-six percent of the faculty responded that " . . . interdisciplinary team teaching had helped increase their appreciation of other health professions faculty" (p. 177). Evaluation data from our first Allied Health Training Grant, Gerontological Initiatives for Visionary Education (GIVE; Kopp Miller, Ishler, & Heater, 1999) has shown that students who participated in the GIVE Project reported an increase in their knowledge of interdisciplinary teamwork and improvement of their attitudes toward working on interdisciplinary teams. The students also agreed that the GIVE Project had a positive impact on their ability to function as effective interdisciplinary team members.

The REAP Project was a direct response to the challenges posed by the preceding national and regional facts. The goal of REAP took into account the problem areas in geriatric education and assessment posed by the literature. To reiterate, the goal of REAP was to educate and prepare a group of allied health educators and students to work effectively as a geriatric health assessment team with a focus on health promotion and disease/dysfunction prevention with community-dwelling, older adults in rural northwest Ohio. The present article describes the implementation of REAP and reports on student outcomes. The interdisciplinary curriculum and field experiences are reviewed and the evaluation method described.

METHOD

Project Implementation

The Rural Elderly Assessment Project was designed to train occupational therapy (OT), physical therapy (PT), physician assistant (PA), and public health (PH) faculty and students to conduct interdisciplinary team health promotion assessments with rural, community-dwelling older adults. The project itself was divided into three distinct phases: Phase I involved faculty and curriculum development; Phase II encompassed the selection and didactic training of student participants; and Phase III involved clinical training in interdisciplinary teams in the community. The project was conducted over the course of three years.

Phase I: Faculty and Curriculum Development. In teaching students to work effectively on interdisciplinary teams, it is essential that faculty be able to model this behavior. One of the major problems in effective interdisciplinary education is the " . . . lack of functioning interdisciplinary clinical role models in teaching and practice" (Baldwin, 1996, p. 182). Although faculty may have experience and training in interdisciplinary teamwork, few full-time academic faculty actually work in interdisciplinary teams on a regular basis. Those who do have regular exposure to clinical interdisciplinary teamwork rarely work on teams comprised solely of professionals from allied health disciplines. For these reasons, much of the first year of REAP was devoted to faculty development.

Faculty representing each of the four disciplines were recruited for the project. The faculty team was comprised of a PA faculty member, a PT faculty member, an OT faculty member, two PH faculty members and the Project Director. The original PH faculty member who was recruited for the project was to be on sabbatical for part of the project so another faculty member from that discipline was involved in order to maintain continuity for the discipline over the course of the project. The Project Director was a psychologist/gerontologist but also a member of the OT faculty.

The REAP faculty team met regularly throughout the first year of the project. The team also participated in two extended retreats with a team development consultant, who had experience in training geriatric interdisciplinary teams. In addition to a variety of group development exercises, team development and growth was facilitated through the completion of specific tasks, such as designing the didactic curriculum for students and developing evaluation strategies to measure student outcomes. An external evaluator also met with the faculty team to guide the development of measurable goals and objectives for the project.

Phase II: Didactic Training for Students. The REAP Project Director and faculty team made brief presentations about the project to the incoming classes of OT, PT, PA, and PH students in the Fall semester of 1998. Students were invited to submit applications to be involved in the project. The application process consisted of students writing an essay explaining why they wanted to participate in the project, the benefits that they felt they would receive from participation and the amount of commitment that they would be able to give to the project. Two recommendation letters from faculty members not directly participating in the project indicating their support of the student application also were required. In addition, the student had to have a minimum 3.0 grade point average and not be on academic probation. The REAP faculty team met and reviewed the applications and discussed any concerns. Twenty-seven students applied and all were selected to participate in the project.

The students completed two, 2-credit hour, graduate level independent studies in the Spring semester and Summer semester of 1999. Specific curriculum components of the first independent study included: biological, psychological and sociological aspects of aging; health promotion and disease prevention with older adults; characteristics of the rural elderly, interdisciplinary team training models and skill development; community resources for older adults; and geriatric health assessment.

Following the didactic training received in the first independent study, students were placed in work groups comprised of students and faculty member(s) of their own discipline. These groups met throughout the course of the summer months to develop a discipline-specific assessment tool for use in the health assessment. Once developed, the tools from each discipline were combined into a comprehensive screening instrument. The instrument was reviewed and modified by faculty with the goals of avoiding unnecessary duplication, reducing the overall length of the assessment, and streamlining the assessment process. Faculty also created a form to document the post-screening team discussion and client recommendations.

Phase III: Interdisciplinary Health Assessment Teams. Following the two didactic independent study courses, students began the experiential component of the project. This phase was conducted during the Fall semester and Spring semester of 2000. Again, students signed up for two, 2-credit, graduate level independent studies during this time. Prior to starting Phase III, students were grouped into six interdisciplinary assessment teams. Each team had a student representative from OT, PT, and PA with some teams having more than one student from the same discipline on the team (this was due to the unequal number of students from each discipline who participated in the project). Because only three PH students were involved with the project, each PH student was responsible to two teams. Three faculty members (OT, PT, PA) were selected to serve as Team Leaders for the health assessment teams with each faculty member being responsible for two teams.

Prior to going out into the field, REAP teams conducted practice screenings using simulated patients and local older adult volunteers recruited for this purpose. Students conducted the practice assessments under the close supervision of their faculty Team Leaders, so that faculty could provide students with feedback, direction, and additional training if warranted. The practice assessments also provided an opportunity to refine the assessment process, the screening tools and questions, the post-assessment team discussion procedures, and the client feedback session process. After the practice sessions were complete, recruitment of community-dwelling, rural older adults began.

Except for the practice sessions, all clients were recruited from rural areas in northwest Ohio. Prior to the beginning of Phase III, the Project Director contacted and formed a relationship with the Care-A-Van Project, a mobile family resource clinic that operates in rural northwest Ohio. Care-A-Van staff and the Project Director identified a variety of community-based sites (e.g., churches, senior centers, VFW halls) that would serve as recruitment locations for the health screenings. The Care-A-Van staff determined that the chosen sites represented the most underserved areas within the county. Assessments were performed within the Care-A-Van clinic and in space designated by the community-based sites. Follow-up visits were conducted at the community-based sites. Through the use of brochures, flyers and word of mouth, the Care-A-Van staff conducted recruitment of older adult participants with help from site representatives. The brochures and flyers outlined the goal of the project, the time commitment involved and the potential benefits that the client would receive from participation. In order to participate in the project, the clients had to agree to complete all written materials required of the project and be able to attend both health assessment sessions.

REAP student teams rotated among the different community-based sites served by the Care-A-Van for four of the five months in Phase III of the project. For one month of the project, all teams performed assessments at a rural retirement community. For these assessments, the facility's health promotion coordinator recruited independent living residents of the retirement community using the same brochures and flyers, and space was provided within the facility for the health promotion assessments and follow-up visits.

The following occurred after a client indicated interest in the project. Once a client was interested, a cover letter indicating the entire process of the health assessment sessions and a health intake questionnaire were mailed with a self-addressed stamped envelope. The health intake questionnaire was designed to retrieve basic health and activity information of the client. The health intake questionnaire was mailed back to the Project Secretary prior to the initial visit and the health intake questionnaire was copied and distributed to the appropriate team for their review. At the initial visit, clients took part in a four-part health promotion assessment with each client seeing all four disciplines on a rotating basis. The entire health promotion assessment took about 75 minutes. At any given time, three of the four professionals were conducting assessments on the clients. The students were required to observe the other three professional assessments when they were not conducting their own assessment. After participating in the health promotion assessment, the client was thanked and a one-week follow-up visit was scheduled. The clients also received a variety of patient education materials on health promotion and healthy aging, and additional health promotion items (e.g., oven stick, hot pad, pill organizer) as thank-you gifts for participating in the project. At any time during this process a client was able to withdraw from participation without consequence.

Immediately after all clients were screened, each team met for an interdisciplinary team discussion. During this time, client assessments were reviewed by each discipline and the team developed health promotion recommendations for each client. Patient education materials and community resources needed by the client were also discussed. This information was shared with each client at his/her one-week follow-up visit. One student member of the team and the faculty Team Leader conducted the follow-up visit.

One hundred and two clients participated in the health promotion assessments during Phase III of REAP. This was a 42% increase over the projected 72 clients who would be served during this phase. Nineteen older adults were recruited from the local metropolitan area, 24 older adults were recruited from a senior center site, 38 older adults came from church sites, 15 older adults were recruited from a retirement community, and the remaining six older adults were recruited from a VFW hall.

Evaluation Methods

The REAP Project employed a comprehensive approach to evaluation. An external evaluation consultant worked closely with the Project Director and the REAP Faculty Team from the outset of the project to design and implement evaluation procedures and methods. Data were obtained primarily through the use of surveys and interviews, and data were collected throughout the course of the project.

Evaluation efforts were designed to be both formative and summative in nature. Project faculty and students were surveyed on a routine basis, and feedback regarding different aspects of the project was provided to project participants and administrators. Changes were made when deemed necessary. For example, the team discussion record was modified from a discipline-reporting format to a problem-based reporting format. This enabled all disciplines to comment on problem areas. The impetus for this change came from the student feedback regarding their experience in the team discussion sessions.

Specific methods were employed to examine discrete portions of the project, such as the didactic curriculum for students and the satisfaction of clients served by the project. The evaluation also made use of extensive pre- and post-testing methodology in order to examine the overall effectiveness of this training project. In the present article, we present preliminary data from only one portion of the project evaluation–the pre- and post-test data collected from the student participants. Specific measures are discussed in detail below.

Pre-Test Questionnaire. Prior to the beginning of their didactic training, students completed a questionnaire designed to examine their initial thoughts about the project and to provide baseline data regarding their self-rated skills and knowledge related to older adults, rural culture, and health promotion and assessment. For each area, students rated their current knowledge or skill on a five-point Likert-type rating scale: Poor (1), Fair (2), Good (3), Very Good (4), or Excellent (5). Open-ended questions tapped students' reasons for applying to the project, their expectations regarding what they would learn, and their concerns and suggestions related to how the project would operate.

The questionnaire also contained the 20-item Team Skills Scale (Hepburn, Tsukuda, & Fasser, 1996; as cited in Siegler, Hyer, Fulmer, & Mezey, 1998) developed for use in the John A. Hartford Foundation's Geriatric Interdisciplinary Team Training initiative and used with permission in the present study. The scale is designed to measure respondents' perceptions of their ability to carry out various tasks associated with interdisciplinary teamwork, as well as their general attitudes toward team care, other disciplines in the team setting, and geriatric patient care. Some of the items are specific to working in a geriatric setting (e.g., "Apply your knowledge of geriatric principles for the care of older persons in a team care setting"), while others address more generic team skills (e.g., "Address client issues succinctly in interdisciplinary meetings"). The measure uses a 5-point Likert-type response scale, with respondents rating their skills and attitudes as Poor (1), Fair (2), Good (3), Very Good (4), or Excellent (5). Prior investigations using this scale have shown that the 17 items that specifically address interdisciplinary team skills tend to emerge as a consistent factor, and demonstrate good reliability as a scale (The Team Skills Scale-Modified, alpha = .95 in studies by Miller, Rose, Bass, Ishler, & Moore, 1998, and Rose, Bass, Ishler, Moore, Whitelaw, & Miller, 1999). Analyses in the present study utilized this 17-item scale, and examined the three items (the attitudinal items) individually.

Post-Test Questionnaire. At the conclusion of the project, students completed a post-test questionnaire designed to assess their self-rated skills, knowledge, and attitudes, as well as provide information about their experience in the project. Students again completed specific self-rated knowledge/skill items and the Team Skills Scale. Students were also asked to respond to a variety of open-ended questions regarding the specific skills and knowledge they gained through the project, the benefits they received as a result of their participation, their perceptions of the project strengths, as well as their recommendations for how to improve the project. Other questions tapped students' overall evaluation of the project, including whether or not they would recommend the project to another student. The time lapse between pre- and post-test was approximately 18 months.

Students' responses to each of the open-ended questions on both the pre- and post-test questionnaires were subjected to thematic analysis conducted by the Project Evaluator. Categories were established based on this analysis, and student responses were coded by the Project Evaluator. The resulting categories and response coding were then reviewed by the Project Director, and any points of disagreement were negotiated and resolved. For some open-ended questions, students were asked to give multiple responses (e.g., "List the top three reasons why you applied to participate in the REAP Project"). In coding, if an individual student gave two or more responses that fell into the same thematic category, these responses were grouped, such that the student was counted only once in the total number of students who gave a response falling into that thematic category.

RESULTS

Student Participants

Twenty-seven students applied and were recruited for participation in the project but two students dropped out of the project prior to its completion. Of the 25 students who completed the project, nine were physical therapy students, nine were occupational therapy students, six were physician assistant students and one was a public health student. As a group, the students were predominantly female (84%) with a mean age of 24.56 (*SD* = 3.44) at project completion. All students were of Caucasian origin.

As was previously noted, two students dropped out of the project prior to its completion. It should be noted that these two students differed significantly from the students who completed the project in terms of discipline (both were PH students) and age (mean age = 31.50, *SD* = 2.12). In addition, one of the students who dropped out of the project was of Asian/Pacific Islander descent. Both students stated that job responsibilities contributed to their discontinuation in the project.

Reasons for Participation in the Project

Students were asked to indicate the top three reasons why they applied to participate in the REAP project. Figure 1 shows the percent of students whose responses fell in each thematic response category. Over three-quarters of students (76%) indicated that they had interest in, enjoyed working with, or wanted to learn more about older adults. As one PA student stated, "I believe there is a need for better understanding of the elderly and thought I'd be part of the solution."

A significant number of students (72%) indicated an interest in interdisciplinary team training and a desire to learn more about the other disciplines. Over half (60%) reported that they applied to participate in the project because of an interest in working with rural populations or obtaining experience in a rural setting. Several students listed factors such as an interest in the health promotion and health assessment focus of the project (16%) and the opportunity to advocate for their profession within the project (16%). A few students (12%) indicated that they thought their participation in the project would make them more marketable upon graduation. Other responses included receiving graduate credit, having an opportunity for general professional growth, and a desire for different clinical experiences.

Student Knowledge, Skills, and Attitudes

At the conclusion of the project, students were asked to list up to three specific skills or knowledge areas that they gained as a result of their participation in REAP. Figure 2 shows the percent of students who reported skill/knowledge gains in each response category. The majority of students (92%) reported gaining interdisciplinary team skills or knowledge related to working with the other disciplines. For example, a PA student reported gaining "Knowledge of the other disciplines' skills

FIGURE 1. Reasons Students Applied to Participate in Project

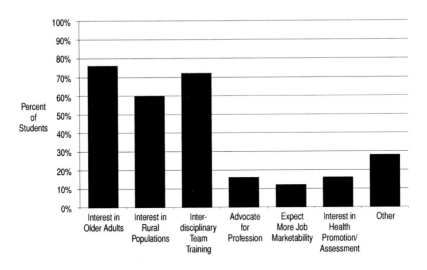

and what they contribute to the health care of the patient." Another PA student indicated, "I now know what 'interdisciplinary' means and how to carry out a meeting, etc., with that in mind." An OT student reported, "I truly understand the benefits of an interdisciplinary team."

Over half (60%) of students reported specific gains in knowledge or skills related to working with older adults, such as "Increased sensitivity to the needs of older adults." A good number of students (40%) indicated that they gained or improved their general clinical skills, such as the "ability to give feedback to clients and information to promote health" or "interviewing skills." Sixteen percent of students reported specific skills or knowledge related to working with rural populations or in a rural environment. Other skills and knowledge gains reported by students included non-specific skills such as "time management," and "communication skills," as well as general professional development (e.g., "confidence in my abilities" and "patience, patience, and more patience").

T-tests were conducted to examine changes in the knowledge, skill, and attitude domains that were specifically targeted by the project. A total of 10 planned comparisons were made. In order to control for the increased risk of a Type I error, a Bonferroni correction was used. The resulting t-statistic for each comparison was regarded as significant only if the associated probability was less than .005.

FIGURE 2. Skill and Knowledge Areas Gained by Student Participants

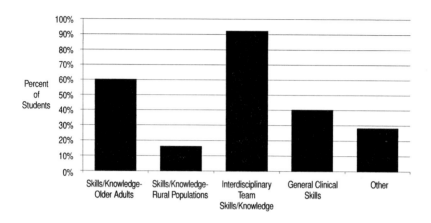

Table 1 presents the results of these comparisons for students' self-rated knowledge and skills related to aging, rural culture, health promotion, and health assessment. In all areas, students' self-rated knowledge and skills showed significant improvement at the end of the project. As a group, students reported significant gains in terms of their knowledge about aging, rural issues, and health promotion. Their post-test ratings also indicated an improvement in interviewing and health assessment skills with older adults. Their self-rated ability to translate health assessment results into interventions was also significantly higher at post-test.

Student pre- and post-test responses to the Team Skills Scale-Modified and three attitudinal measures were analyzed to examine changes. These results are presented in Table 2. Students demonstrated significant improvements in terms of their mean item scores on the Team Skills Scale-Modified. They also reported improvements in their attitudes toward other disciplines and toward practicing in a team care environment. Changes in students' self-reported attitudes toward providing care for the elderly were not significantly different from pre- to post-test.

Overall Evaluation of the Project

Students perceived a number of benefits of having been a participant in REAP. All students identified specific skills or knowledge that they

TABLE 1. Student Self-Rated Skills and Knowlege

	Pre-Test Mean[a] (Std Dev)	Post-Test Mean[a] (Std Dev)	T-test Results[b]
Knowledge about aging and older adults	2.68 (.80)	4.16 (.47)	$t = 8.06$, $df = 24$*
Knowledge about rural issues	2.64 (1.35)	3.96 (.74)	$t = 5.77$, $df = 24$*
Knowledge about health promotion/ disease prevention	2.68 (.75)	4.24 (.78)	$t = 8.12$, $df = 24$*
Skills in interviewing and communicating with older adults	2.68 (.90)	4.46 (.59)	$t = 7.00$, $df = 23$*
Skills in conducting health assessments with older adult clients	1.88 (.78)	4.28 (.61)	$t = 12.00$, $df = 24$*
Ability to translate health assessment results into client-oriented interventions	1.80 (.76)	4.28 (.74)	$t = 12.34$, $df = 24$*

[a] Ratings used a 5-point Likert-type scale (1 = Poor, 2 = Fair, 3 = Good, 4 = Very Good, 5 = Excellent).
[b] 1-tailed, using a Bonferroni correction for the total number of planned comparisons (10).
* $p < .005$

gained as a benefit of participating in the project. Over half (60%) perceived themselves as having received a competitive advantage in the job market as a result of their participation (e.g., "I may be considered as a better candidate for a job because of this experience"). Twenty percent of students indicated that they had developed new friendships and professional relationships through the project. Three students (12%) reported that they had developed or expanded a specific career interest (e.g., working with the elderly, working in a rural setting) through their participation in REAP. Other benefits cited by students included feelings of accomplishment, respect, and appreciation.

Students were asked to identify the specific strengths of REAP. Many students (64%) cited the interdisciplinary nature of the project as a strength. Forty percent mentioned the direct client contact and the real-life, practical skill-building experience provided by the project. Several students (28%) cited the overall design of the project, how the project was organized, or the flexibility and responsiveness of the project as strengths. Sixteen percent of students specifically identified the community outreach provided by the project as a strength. Project faculty and staff and resources available to/provided by the project were

TABLE 2. Student Team Skills and Attitudes

	Pre-Test Mean[a] (Std Dev)	Post-Test Mean[a] (Std Dev)	T-test Results[b]
Team Skills Scale-Modified mean item score	2.97 (.70)	4.21 (.42)	$t = 8.45$, $df = 24$*
Attitude toward other disciplines working in the team setting	3.88 (.60)	4.56 (.51)	$t = 4.92$, $df = 24$*
Attitude toward providing care to the elderly	4.32 (.63)	4.64 (.49)	$t = 2.32$, $df = 24$
Attitude about practicing in a team care environment	4.12 (.67)	4.68 (.56)	$t = 3.65$, $df = 24$*

[a] Ratings used a 5-point Likert-type scale (1 = Poor, 2 = Fair, 3 = Good, 4 = Very Good, 5 = Excellent).
[b] 1-tailed, using a Bonferroni correction for the total number of planned comparisons (10).
* $p < .005$

cited by sixteen percent of students. Two students (8%) mentioned that they perceived the project as geared toward their specific learning needs. As one PT student put it, "This program was geared to pick up at an appropriate level for my education and advance me to the next level." Other strengths cited by students included the opportunity to meet and work with other students, the enthusiasm of project participants, and the uniqueness of the project.

Students provided specific suggestions for how to improve the project. Most suggestions involved making modifications to the logistics of the clinical experience, such as picking sites that were closer to the college to eliminate driving time, or improved communication regarding travel arrangements. Twenty-eight percent of students recommended increasing the scope of the project to include more students and more client assessments. Several students also suggested that the interdisciplinary teams be created earlier, to provide them with more time to work together and grow as a team. Other suggestions for improvement revolved around decreasing the survey burden for evaluation and changes to the order or emphasis of team-training activities.

When asked for their overall evaluation of the project, students provided favorable ratings. On a scale of 1 (Poor) to 5 (Excellent), students' mean rating was 4.24 ($SD = .66$), in the Good-Excellent range.

Fully 100% of the students indicated that they would recommend participating in REAP to another student. Student comments included:

It was a great opportunity to enhance my knowledge of interdisciplinary teams, other allied health professionals, and increase my confidence level.–PT student

It makes you really decide how you would like to function in the future and makes you more marketable.–PA student

I believe it's an invaluable clinical experience in geriatrics and with an interdisciplinary team.–OT student

DISCUSSION

The occupational therapy, physical therapy, physician assistant, and public health students who participated in REAP clearly saw the project as a valuable part of their education. Students signed up for the project because it offered experience with older adult clients, interdisciplinary team training, and exposure to practice in a rural setting. At the conclusion of the project, most students were able to articulate that the project had provided them with specific skills and knowledge related to interdisciplinary teamwork and working with the elderly.

Comparison of student pre- and post-project ratings with respect to their knowledge, skills, and attitudes provides evidence as to the intended impact of the project. Students reported improvements in all but one of the knowledge, skill, and attitude domains that were specifically targeted by the project. Only students' self-rated attitudes toward providing care to the elderly were not significantly different from pre- to post-test. Not surprisingly, students expressed positive attitudes toward the care of older adults prior to their involvement in the project, and their attitudes remained positive after the project was completed.

As perceived by the students, the benefits of participating in the project extended beyond the knowledge and skills they developed. Many students saw themselves as more marketable as a result of the project. Students also reported that the project helped them to make new friends and develop professional relationships they may not have otherwise developed. Several students indicated that involvement in REAP had significantly influenced their career goals and expectations. Perhaps most telling, all of the students said that they would recommend the project to another student.

The significant results obtained from the student evaluation data may have been influenced by the self-report nature of the measures employed. We cannot ignore the possibility that students inflated their post-test ratings in order to justify the extensive time and effort they contributed to the project. One important result does provide evidence to the contrary, however; student attitudes toward providing care to the elderly were not significantly improved at the conclusion of the project. If students inflated their post-test ratings, one would expect the inflation to be relatively uniform, not selective.

Limitations

The present paper reports on only a portion of the evaluation data gathered during the project, and is limited to the subjective evaluations of the student participants. It is possible that students' knowledge, attitudes, and skills did not improve, or did not improve as dramatically as they believed (or indicated) they did. Alternatively, it is possible that improvements did occur, but that the REAP project was not the causative factor in these changes. Student perceptions of the project and its value may also differ markedly from the perceptions of others involved in the project. As previously mentioned, data were collected from REAP faculty, elderly clients who participated in the interdisciplinary health promotion assessments, and project partners in the community. Data were also collected from the peers of the REAP students, allowing for comparison of REAP students to their counterparts who completed their traditional discipline-specific curricula. Analysis of, and comparison with, these other data will allow for a more sophisticated and complete examination of the impact of this project.

The attrition of the two public health students from the project deserves discussion. Both PH students dropped out of the project during Phase III. This attrition may have been attributable to several factors. First, there appeared to be an incompatibility between the time demands of the project and these students' schedules. As the project evolved, the Project Director and Team Leaders were able to successfully negotiate adjustments to student class schedules and fieldwork practica placements. Such negotiations were more difficult with the PH program, as it is a joint degree program between three institutions of higher education in the area. In addition, the extra time required by the REAP project in Phase III, especially when factoring in travel time to and from remote locations, seemed especially burdensome to the PH students. Another factor complicating the involvement of PH students was a lack of clarity regarding their role in the assessment process. At the outset of the project, faculty saw PH as occupying a consultative role in the health promotion assessments–they would be brought in when it was suspected that a client could benefit from having a consultation with PH. In reality, the role of PH evolved and expanded as the project continued. It is possible that greater clarification regarding the role of PH and the expectations of PH students might have prevented their attrition from the project.

The results of this evaluation are strengthened by the use of a prospective study design, thus eliminating retrospective bias in student ratings of their knowledge, skills, and attitudes. In addition, investigators took substantial steps to minimize the possibility of type I error and employed a conservative alpha level for the statistical comparisons of students' pre- and post-test ratings. Although the results of this evaluation cannot be generalized beyond the students who participated in REAP, they do provide suggestions for potential project replication and recommendations for the interdisciplinary training of allied health students.

Lessons Learned and Recommendations for Allied Health Interdisciplinary Team Training

It is often difficult to develop and implement interdisciplinary team training within a given organization. Barriers do exist. To the extent that such barriers can be identified and articulated prior to project implementation, increased success in interdisciplinary training is more likely. From an administrative perspective, the success of such training is enhanced if key players are supportive of the project from the onset and logistical and scheduling concerns are identified in the beginning of the project. The key players of REAP were the administration and the faculty and students who were ultimately involved in the project. By keeping administrators informed about the project (from concept to implementation), the possibility of success was increased. Specific requests that had to be made to administrators throughout the project were handled efficiently and effectively because they were kept informed of how REAP was progressing throughout all phases.

In order to solicit support from faculty and students, both groups were given incentives for participating in the project. The success of REAP was dependent upon involving faculty and training them to mentor and guide the interdisciplinary teams. With permission from administration, the faculty involved in REAP were able to use their time in REAP as part of their faculty development. A portion of the faculty member's salary was also covered by the grant as well as a portion of the faculty's travel to conferences and workshops that they attended as part of REAP. Incentives for students were also available. Graduate credit and a graduate certificate, which was awarded after completion of the project, enabled students to be supportive of the project. In fact, many students reported that this was the reason why they chose to participate in the project at the onset.

Scheduling and logistical problems of the project did occur throughout all Phases. In an effort to minimize the impact of these barriers, the REAP faculty, Project Director and Project Evaluator spent a considerable amount of time discussing different ways to implement the project if certain scheduling barriers could not be worked out. This planning time proved invaluable when the conflicts arose and kept the project on schedule.

It is the opinion of the authors that a variety of training methods improves the overall interdisciplinary team training experience for both the faculty and students. The didactic training provided to students in Phase II of the Project created an opportunity for students to develop a shared understanding of the distinct roles and responsibilities of each discipline, as well as those roles and responsibilities that are shared across disciplines. By involving students in work groups charged with developing the discipline-specific components of the health assessment tools, students were afforded an opportunity to enhance their confidence in the knowledge and practice of their own disciplines.

The instructional methods and skill development strategies employed in REAP may help direct allied health educators who are struggling to provide students with both strong disciplinary instruction and instruction in interdisciplinary teamwork. This "dual socialization" (Clark, 1997) is necessary in order for students to develop identities as both individual practitioners and team members.

The REAP project also demonstrated the value of learning and practicing interdisciplinary team skills out in the community. By participating in an actual clinical situation that provided a service to needy clients, students learned to respect the contribution of other disciplines and to appreciate the sociocultural experiences of the clients they served. Similar findings have been demonstrated in other interdisciplinary training projects that have taken students out into underserved communities to perform health promotion assessments and evaluations, for example, the Tillery Project in rural North Carolina (Wittman, Conner-Kerr, Templeton, & Velde, 1999).

Outcome data from students indicate that the REAP project was a positive learning experience that provided them with a solid foundation for interdisciplinary practice with geriatric clients. The project also provided a service to rural, community-dwelling older adults. REAP was a successful partnership among an academic health center, a mobile health clinic, and community-based sites.

AUTHOR'S NOTE

This publication was made possible by grant number #1-D37-AH-00644 from the Bureau of Health Professions, Health Resources and Services Administration. Its contents are solely the responsibility of the authors and do not necessarily represent the official views of the Bureau of Health Professions.

The authors would like to express their appreciation to the REAP faculty team (Farhang Akbar, PhD, Michael Bisesi, PhD, Catherine Hornbeck, MS, PT, Martin Rice, PhD, OTR/L, Patricia Francis, MS), the students who participated in the project, and those members of the local community who helped ensure the project's success.

REFERENCES

American Association of Retired Persons and Administration on Aging (1998). *A profile of older Americans.* Washington, DC: AARP Fulfillment.

Area Office on Aging of Northwestern Ohio, Inc. (1994). *A strategic plan for programs and services for northwest Ohio's older population.* Toledo, OH: Author.

Baldwin, D. C. (1996). Some historical notes on interdisciplinary and interprofessional education and practice in health care in the USA. *Journal of Interprofessional Care, 10 (2),* 173-187.

Buck, M.M., Tilson, E.R., & Andersen, J.C. (1999). Implementation and evaluation of an interdisciplinary health professions core curriculum. *Journal of Allied Health, 28,* 174-178.

Carstensen, L.L., Edelstein, B.A., & Dornbrand, L. (1996). *The practical handbook of clinical gerontology.* Thousand Oaks, CA: Sage Publications.

Clark, P.G. (1997). Values in health care professional socialization: Implications for geriatric education in interdisciplinary teamwork. *Gerontologist, 37 (4),* 441-451.

Kopp Miller, B., Ishler, K.J., & Heater, S. (1999). Gerontological initiatives for visionary education project: Interdisciplinary training for occupational and physical therapy students. *Gerontology & Geriatrics Education, 19 (3),* 21-37.

Krout, J.A. (1994). *Providing community-based services to the rural elderly.* Thousand Oaks, CA: Sage Publications.

Krout, J.A. (1998). Services and service delivery in rural environments. In R.T. Coward & J. A. Krout (Eds.), *Aging in rural settings: Life circumstances and distinctive features* (pp. 247-266). New York: Springer Publishing Company.

Miller, B., Rose, J. H., Bass, D., Ishler, K. J., & Moore, S. M. (1998, November). Effects of an interdisciplinary team training pilot program. Poster presented at the annual meeting of the Gerontological Society of America, Philadelphia, PA.

Mockenhaupt, R. E. & Muchow, J. A. (1994). Disease and disability prevention and health promotion for rural elders. In J. A. Krout (Ed.), *Providing community-based services to the rural elderly* (pp. 183-201). Thousand Oaks, CA: Sage Publications.

Northwest Ohio Health Planning, Inc. (1997). *Community-based health resources plan for Health Service Area 4.* Toledo, OH: Northwest Ohio Health Planning, Inc.

O'Neil, E.H. & the Pew Health Professions Commission (1998). *Recreating health professional practice for a new century.* San Francisco: Pew Health Professions Commission.

Pew Health Professions Commission (1995). *Critical challenges: Revitalizing the health professions for the twenty-first century.* San Francisco, CA: Author.

Pfeiffer, E. (1999). Basic principles of working with older patients: An up-date. *Gerontology & Geriatrics Education, 20 (1),* 3-13.

Rose, J. H., Bass, D. M., Ishler, K. J., Moore, S. M., Whitelaw, N., & Miller, B. (1999, November). Team training: Trainee characteristics affect team care attitudes and skills. Poster presented at the annual meeting of the Gerontological Society of America, San Francisco, CA.

Scripps Gerontology Center (1990). *Ohio long term care research.* Oxford, OH: Author.

Siegler, E. L., Hyer, K., Fulmer, T., & Mezey, M. (1998). Developed for the John A. Hartford GITT Project. Published source: Appendix B, Section I: Core Measures for the GITT Program (pp. 259-277), in E.L. Siegler, K. Hyer, T. Fulmer, & M. Mezey (Eds.), *Geriatric interdisciplinary team training.* New York: Springer.

U.S. Department of Health and Human Services (1990). *Healthy people 2000: National health promotion and disease prevention objectives.* Washington, DC: Author.

U.S. Department of Health and Human Services (1996). *A national agenda for geriatric education: White papers.* Washington, DC: Author.

Wittman, P., Conner-Kerr, T., Templeton, M.S., &Velde, B. (1999). The Tillery Project: An experience in an interdisciplinary rural health care service setting. *Physical & Occupational Therapy in Geriatrics, 17 (1),* 17-28.

Physical Therapy and Occupational Therapy: Partners in Rehabilitation for Persons with Movement Impairments

David L. Nelson, PhD, OTR
Daniel J. Cipriani, MEd, PT
Julie J. Thomas, PhD, OTR

SUMMARY. The professions of physical therapy and occupational therapy have legitimate roles in the restoration of human movement in the rehabilitation process. This paper first presents a physical therapy perspective on changing trends in therapeutic exercise. Recent trends in physical therapy reflect a shift away from isolating patterns of movement and open kinetic chain exercises toward a new emphasis on functional patterns of movement and closed kinetic chain exercises. Rehabilitation of persons with hip fracture is used as an example of these shifting trends. Next, the paper presents an occupational therapy perspective. Occupational therapy's historical emphasis on the use of naturalistic occupations as the context for therapeutic exercise is described. Theoretical advantages of occupationally embedded movement are listed, and recent

---

David L. Nelson is Professor, Department of Occupational Therapy, Medical College of Ohio, Toledo, OH 43614.

Daniel J. Cipriani is Assistant Professor, Department of Physical Therapy, Medical College of Ohio, Toledo, OH 43614.

Julie J. Thomas is Associate Professor and Chair, Department of Occupational Therapy, Medical College of Ohio, Toledo, OH 43614.

[Haworth co-indexing entry note]: "Physical Therapy and Occupational Therapy: Partners in Rehabilitation for Persons with Movement Impairments." Nelson, David L., Daniel J. Cipriani, and Julie J. Thomas. Co-published simultaneously in *Occupational Therapy in Health Care* (The Haworth Press, Inc.) Vol. 15, No. 3/4, 2001, pp. 35-57; and: *Interprofessional Collaboration in Occupational Therapy* (ed: Stanley Paul, and Cindee Q. Peterson) The Haworth Press, Inc., 2001, pp. 35-57. Single or multiple copies of this article are available for a fee from The Haworth Document Delivery Service [1-800-HAWORTH, 9:00 a.m. - 5:00 p.m. (EST). E-mail address: getinfo@haworthpressinc.com].

35

research in support of naturalistic occupations is summarized. Physical therapy and occupational therapy are distinct professions with autonomous outlooks and terminologies, but the responsibilities of physical therapists and occupational therapists potentially overlap in the restoration of movement. Suggestions are made for interdisciplinary teamwork whereby the holistically considered welfare of the patient is always the primary concern of all therapists. *[Article copies available for a fee from The Haworth Document Delivery Service: 1-800-HAWORTH. E-mail address: <getinfo@haworthpressinc.com> Website: <http://www.HaworthPress.com> © 2001 by The Haworth Press, Inc. All rights reserved.]*

KEYWORDS. Function, task-oriented movement, occupationally embedded movement, hip fracture

A PHYSICAL THERAPY PERSPECTIVE

A Traditional Emphasis on Pathomechanics

Traditional physical therapy exercises address the specific pathomechanics involved in dysfunction. With traditional rehabilitation, physical therapists apply exercise approaches that tend to isolate the area of dysfunction and implement exercises that address the specific deficiency of the involved joint or muscle. For example, in the case of rehabilitation for persons with hip fracture, physical therapists address specific issues of hip range of motion and muscle strength around the hip complex. Exercises such as the prone hip extensions, supine straight leg raising, isometric setting exercises of the gluteus maximus, and side lying hip abduction exercises are a few examples of the exercise programs that dominate traditional lower extremity (LE) rehabilitation (Russell & Palmieri, 1996). Moreover, because individuals perform these exercises in a non-weight bearing position, with the distal segment (i.e., the foot) free to move, physical therapists have applied the label of open kinetic chain (OKC) to these exercises (Fitzgerald, 1997; Yack, Collins, & Whieldon, 1993; Fu, Woo, & Irrgang, 1992).

These isolating exercises focus on the measured deficiency of the LE. As in the above example of the hip fracture rehabilitation plan, exercise programs attempt to restore strength and mobility of the involved hip joint. As strength and mobility improve, the traditional physical therapy program moves individuals toward weight bearing exercises such as gait training, stair climbing, and transfer training (Russell & Palmieri, 1996). However, individuals need to first demonstrate adequate performance of the OKC exercises before being progressed to the weight bearing program.

A Shift Toward Function and Closed Kinetic Chain (CKC) Exercises

The assumptions behind traditional approaches are often difficult to question, but it is now clear that strategies in physical therapy have undergone a gradual shift. This shift is from a focus on isolated exercises toward a focus on integrated exercises (Duscha, Cipriani, & Roberts, 1999; Jenkins, Bronner, & Mangine, 1997). Physical therapists have developed a greater appreciation for functionally oriented exercises, compared with joint or muscle-oriented exercise approaches. In other words, physical therapy for lower extremity rehabilitation places a great emphasis on exercises that incorporate weight bearing and that mimic specific lower extremity tasks (e.g., stair stepping exercises, squats, lunges, standing balance drills, etc.). These "functional" exercises are in addition to the traditional joint and muscle isolation exercises. Thus, rehabilitation, from the physical therapy perspective, can be viewed as a continuum which progresses from least functional (mostly joint- or muscle-isolating) toward more functional and integrated movements (mostly CKC movements) (Gray, 1993).

By the end of the 1980s and into the early 1990s, physical therapy professionals began questioning the role of isolated exercises (Cipriani & Vermillion, 1995; Gray, 1993). Continuing education courses and research began to address the issue of exercise efficacy and exercise specificity (Morrissey, Harman, & Johnson, 1995; Gray, 1993). Closed kinetic chain exercises began to gain in popularity as the primary source of exercise. Research supported the notion that weight bearing exercises such as the leg squat and step-up exercise could be as effective for gaining strength and mobility as the more traditional OKC version (e.g., knee extensions, hip extensions).

Augustsson, Esko, Thomee, and Svantsesson (1998) demonstrated that CKC exercises are more effective for strengthening the quadriceps muscles than OKC. They compared the traditional standing squat exercise (CKC exercise group) with the traditional seated knee extension and hip adduction exercises (OKC exercise group). Post-test strength results increased for both groups of subjects; however, the group performing standing squat exercises demonstrated greater strength gains than the seated exercise group (31% gain vs. 13% gain, $p < .05$). They further noted that CKC exercises more closely reproduced the function of the quadriceps (i.e., controlling knee flexion in stance) than OKC exercises.

In addition, research supports the notion that CKC exercises may better prepare an individual for return to normal tasks of daily living, compared with OKC exercise (Anderson, Gieck, Perrin et al., 1991; Blackburn & Morrissey, 1998; and Worrell, Borchert, Erner et al., 1993). Worrell, Borchert, Erner et al. examined the effects of a four-week progressive strengthening program of the lower extremity in healthy individuals. The program consisted of a common CKC exercise, the lateral step up/down exercise. Subjects performed multiple repetitions of stepping up/down on a step while holding a prescribed amount of weight in each hand for external resistance. The weight component was increased gradually over the course of the strengthening program using the daily adjusted progressive resistance exercise protocol. All subjects were pre-tested and post-tested for OKC strength using an isokinetic dynamometer as well as for functional strength using hop tests and step tests. At the conclusion of the training program, all subjects demonstrated significant gains in hopping abilities and stepping abilities ($p < .05$). The investigators did not observe significant gains with the OKC strength testing. Finally, studies by Greenberger and Paterno (1995) and Anderson, Gieck, Perrin et al. (1991) failed to show any strong relationships between OKC strength testing and functional performance abilities.

A Continuum of Function

Physical therapists now classify functional exercises on a continuous scale. OKC exercises represent one end of the scale, typically the lower end of function, while CKC exercises represent the opposite end of the scale, namely more functional. Essentially, although the prone hip extension exercise does not replicate any typical movement of function, it is on the continuum of function. This exercise elicits muscle effort from the gluteus maximus and hamstrings and requires hip movement through the available range. However, a squatting exercise also elicits effort from the gluteus maximus and hamstrings and requires hip movement through the available range. In addition, the squatting exercise also requires movement from the ankles, knees, and pelvis, as well as effort from the posterior calf muscles (e.g., gastrocnemius and soleus), the quadriceps, and the back extensors. Thus, the squatting exercise integrates the entire lower extremity rather than isolating the hip joint. Physical therapists consider this CKC exercise to be more functional than the hip extension exercise, which does not resemble any typical daily task. In addition, the squat exercise closely resembles the components of motion involved in the process of sit-to-stand and stand-to-sit. Table 1 illustrates common CKC exercises, and the functional tasks they replicate.

A Task-Oriented Approach

Recently, rehabilitation specialists have stretched the continuum of function even further. The advocacy of task-oriented behaviors in place of rote-type exercises has expanded the definition of function for lower

TABLE 1. Lower Extremity Exercises Simulating Function

Exercise	Functional Simulation
Squats	Replicates movements encountered during gait, stair climbing/descending, and sit-to-stand/stand-to-sit
Lunges	Replicates movements encountered during initial loading in gait/can be performed in sagital, frontal, and transverse planes
Automated Stair Climbers	Replicates forces similar to stair climbing
Biomechanical Ankle Platform System (BAPS board)	Replicates transverse plane forces of the entire lower extremity
Cross-Country Ski Machines	Replicates saggital plane forces, without major ground reaction forces
Versa Climbers	Replicates forces similar to stair climbing, and ladder climbing, including reciprocal arm motions
Treadmills	Allows forward, backward, and sideward walking for gait training in the clinical setting
Total Gym Incline Boards	One and two legged squats to replicate forces similar to standing squats in a protected position

extremity rehabilitation. Task-oriented behaviors involve the supervised practice of actual activities of daily living (ADL) and instrumental activities of daily living (IADL). While task-oriented behaviors have always been implemented in the lower extremity rehabilitation program, therapists have viewed this component of the program as a separate stage of rehabilitation, and not typically as a component of the exercise session. In addition, physical therapists have typically reserved this portion of the therapy program for the final stages of a person's rehabilitation.

The dilemma facing rehabilitation specialists continues to be efficacy of the rehabilitation strategy. While defining the term function continues to evolve, placing rehabilitation strategies along a continuum seems to work well. Unfortunately, therapists are not fully sure which portion of the continuum is best suited for rehabilitation of the lower extremity. Recent research comparing OKC methods to CKC methods supports the CKC approach, mainly because weight-bearing exercises are as effective at making strength gains and better replicate function (Worrell, Borchert, Erner et al., 1993; Augustsson, Esko, Thomee, & Svantsesson, 1998; Fitzgerald, 1997). Research is not available comparing CKC exercises (rote exercises) with task-oriented behaviors (functional activities) in terms of overall rehabilitation and preparing an individual for return to life.

Advocates for the task-oriented behaviors might argue that this approach is more efficient from a time management standpoint. Individuals practice the behaviors they will face in their home or work environment, from the very beginning of rehabilitation, optimizing the time spent during rehabilitation by focusing on the functional demands of the individual. In addition, practicing these tasks should result in strength and mobility gains for the involved area of dysfunction. Theoretically, this approach can be defended by the concept of exercise specificity, or specificity of training (Morrissey, Harman, & Johnson, 1995; Brotzman & Head, 1996).

Morrissey, Harman, and Johnson (1995) performed a comprehensive literature review regarding the topic of exercise specificity. By definition, this concept refers to the fact that the mode of exercise dictates the physiological adaptations of the human body. In other words, the body will gain the way it is trained. Performing an exercise at slow speeds (e.g., 30 degrees per second) will improve an individual's ability to move at this slow speed, but it may not improve an individual's ability to perform the same movement at a high speed. For example, an individual wishing to improve her ability to run sprints will not yield substantial improvements if she trains at a slow-paced jog. Morrissey, Harman, and Johnson demonstrated that this concept of exercise specificity carries over to most exercise approaches. Exercise specificity plays a role in the range of motion that an individual exercises through, the speed of the motion, the type of muscle action (i.e., eccentric, concentric, isometric), and the complexity of the motion involved. Thus, advocates of task-oriented exercises argue that the best way to rehabilitate an individual to perform specific tasks is to have that person perform the specific tasks as part of the rehabilitation process. Simply performing traditional muscle strengthening may not prepare an individual to use that muscle during complex activities of daily living.

For example, research on ankle instability illustrates the need for task-specific training. Several investigations demonstrated that a sole focus on rehabilitating lost muscle strength is insufficient to improve lost balance skills with individuals suffering ankle sprains (Lentell, Baas, Lopez et al., 1995; Rozzi, Lephart, Sterner, & Kuligowski, 1999). According to Lentell, Baas, Lopez et al. (1995), regaining ankle strength following injury did not guarantee a return of normal balance and position sense within the injured ankle. Apparently, in order to restore balance abilities, rehabilitation needed to address balance deficits specifically. This was supported by Rozzi, Lephart, Sterner, and Kuligowski (1999). Their investigation evaluated the effects of a balance training program on the standing balance measures of individuals with functionally unstable ankles. Following a four-week training program exclusively limited to balance training exercises, subjects with previous reports of ankle instability demonstrated significant improvements in their reports of ankle stability. In addition, physical measures of standing balance improved significantly following the balance training program.

Rote Exercise versus a Task Orientation

While task-oriented exercises make sense intuitively, advocates of rote type exercises might argue that CKC allows the rehabilitation specialist to challenge an individual at a level far greater than that individual will face in the home or work environment (Augustsson, Esko, Thomee, & Svantsesson, 1998; Cipriani & Vermillion, 1995). For example, performing multiple repetitions of knee squats typically exceeds the amount of work needed to rise from a chair or to sit. By performing rote exercises, the rehabilitation specialist not only prepares the individual for the normal functional stresses, but also prepares the individual for the unexpected stresses. These unexpected stresses might include carrying packages up a flight of stairs, or having enough strength and mobility to recover from a near slip and fall. Unless an individual performs the task-oriented behaviors under numerous situations and with numerous repetitions, this approach may not fully prepare the individual for the unexpected stresses of life.

On the other hand, there is research support for the rote exercise approach. Research with the elderly supports the notion that rote exercises contribute to functional abilities (Judge, Underwood, & Gennosa, 1993; Cress, Buchner, Questad et al., 1999; Judge, Lindsey, Underwood, & Winsemius, 1993; Ades, Ballor, Ashikaga et al., 1996). For example, Cress, Buchner, Questad et al. (1999) studied the effects of a standard rote exercise program for total body strength and endurance. They evaluated two groups of healthy elderly individuals. One group performed exercises while the control group engaged in no exercise. Exercises included traditional free weight dumbbell exercises, stair stepping machines, leg press machines, and cuff weight exercises. Following a six-month training program, the exercising group reported significant gains in function, as measured by the Continuous Scale–Physical Performance Functional Performance test. In addition, this group demonstrated significant gains in maximal oxygen consumption (11%) and muscle strength (33%). The Cress, Buchner, Questad et al. (1999) investigation supports the results of previous investigations looking at the impact of lower extremity strengthening on function in the elderly. Studies by Ades, Douglas, Ballor et al. (1996) and Judge, Underwood, and Gennosa (1993) have also demonstrated that strength training of the lower extremities significantly improved walking endurance and walking speed in elderly populations. In summary, rote exercise can indeed improve certain functions. However, it is an open question for research as to the relative efficacy of rote exercise and a task-oriented approach.

AN OCCUPATIONAL THERAPY PERSPECTIVE

Historical Context

The idea of embedding therapeutic exercise within culturally defined occupations has been an organizing principle of occupational therapy since the founding of the profession. In 1919, Bird T. Baldwin (p. 5), Director of Occupational Therapy and Chief Psychologist at Walter Reed Hospital, stated: "Occupational therapy is based on the principle that the best type of remedial exercise is that which requires a series of specific voluntary movements involved in the ordinary trades and occupations, physical training, play, or the daily routine activities of life." Susan Johnson (1920, p. 2), one of the founders of the profession of occupational therapy, gave the following example of occupationally embedded movement: "Patient after patient . . . with little or no control of arm or leg . . . became so interested in weaving a rug . . . that he forgot his disability and unconsciously employed the disabled member; and so gained strength and courage for other occupation with surprising rapidity." Many other examples of the same principle are documented in Dunton's important text of occupational therapy (Dunton, 1928). The idea of embedding therapeutic exercise within occupation might well have been a reason that the fledgling profession of occupational therapy first became involved in what is today called "physical disabilities."

A Conceptual Framework for Therapeutic Occupation

A modern conceptual framework for therapeutic occupation is depicted in Figure 1 (Nelson, 1988; 1994). In this framework, occupation is conceptualized as the relationship between an occupational form and an occupational performance. Occupational therapists synthesize or create occupational forms (objective circumstances with sociocultural and physical dimensions) that guide or elicit a person's occupational performance (doing, behaving). The person, through his or her unique developmental structure, can find meaning in the occupational form, which leads to purposes for engaging in an occupational performance.

Occupation is therapeutic when the patient's occupational performance results in adaptations to the developmental structure (positive changes in sensorimotor, cognitive, or psychosocial abilities). Occupational performance may also result in an impact on subsequent occupational forms (e.g., materials are changed, a meal is prepared, one's clothing is put on).

Naturalistic Occupation and Occupationally Embedded Movement

In occupationally embedded movement, the occupational form is a culturally recognizable situation (e.g., a dice game, plants that need watering). The occupational form is synthesized (set up, or structured) in such a way as to be meaningful and purposeful to the individual, while requiring a therapeutic occupational performance (pattern of voluntary movement). For example, the dice game might be part of the patient's favorite game prior to experiencing a fall and a hip fracture. If placed on a 40″ high table, the game materials can elicit the occupational perfor-

FIGURE 1. In Occupationally Embedded Movement, the Occupational Thera-
pist Collaborates with the Patient in Synthesizing a Naturalistic Occupational
Form that Will Have Meaning and Purpose to the Patient, and that Will Lead to
Voluntary Occupational Performance and Beneficial Adaptations.

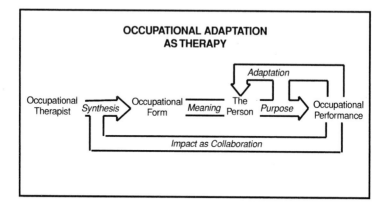

mance of prolonged standing. The patient is able to see her own impact
on the materials over the course of the game (winning the game might
be possible if there is another person in the occupational form). A therapeutic adaptation is the increased standing tolerance developed as a
consequence of playing the game. For another example, plants in the
hospital lobby (occupational form) provide the opportunity for meaningful, purposeful occupational performances leading to multiple adaptations, including increased dynamic standing balance and increased
safety awareness as the patient negotiates obstacles in the occupational
form. The same principle of occupationally embedded exercise could
be applied to a program for upper extremity strengthening for the
deconditioned patient with a hip fracture.

A problem is that therapists often do not have ready access to totally
naturalistic home-based and community-based settings. Therefore, therapists frequently rely on simulations of everyday settings (e.g., the patient's hospital room, the "OT kitchen," or the hospital lobby and gift
shop). In a simulation, some of the naturalistic features are present,
while some aspects of the occupational form are artificial. For example,
the dice game materials are naturalistic, but a table set up in the patient's
hospital room (with interruptions for nursing care) is part of an artificial, or atypical, setting. Simulations may be near-naturalistic or far-
from-naturalistic. An example of a far-from-naturalistic simulation is

the use of one-pound weights as substitutes for common household items to be stacked on shelves. Here, the therapist's words cue the patient to the idea that "reorganizing the kitchen cabinets" is being simulated. Simulations are effective to the extent that the patient finds meaning in them, leading to purposeful and beneficial performance. Some persons appreciate simulations; some do not. A principle of occupational therapy is to tinker with the occupational form and to consult with the patient about the occupational form until maximal meaning and purpose is achieved, given practical constraints.

Nelson and Peterson (1989) described therapeutic situations as on a continuum, from total naturalism to rote patterns of exercise. In rote exercise, materials involve specialized therapy equipment not otherwise found in daily life, and the therapist's instructions do not suggest everyday, recognizable occupations. Near and far simulations are at various points on the continuum. A special case of a far simulation is the use of imagery with little or no naturalistic materials. For example, a patient might be asked to reach up to pick imaginary apples, or to lean down to pick up imaginary coins from the floor (Riccio, Nelson, & Bush, 1990). Here the important part of the occupational form is the speech of the therapist, and the patient must assign meaning to the words based on past experience. This kind of imagery to promote occupational therapy has been used for over 90 years in occupational therapy. For example, Cohn (1906) suggested that imagery about rowing a boat could elicit therapeutic patterns of performance in patients with mental illness.

Theoretical Advantages and Disadvantages of Naturalistic Occupation

Theoretically (Nelson & Peterson, 1989), what are the possible arguments in favor of the naturalistic as opposed to the rote end of the continuum?

1. In naturalistic occupation, the patient can see the results of his own efforts, because the environment is typically impacted. For example, the patient can see that the car has been polished because of vigorous work. In contrast, a piece of exercise equipment is unchanged at the end of exercise.

2. In naturalistic occupation, the patient can judge the success or failure of her performance in terms of personal and sociocultural criteria. For example, the patient can see that she is able to make part of the bed, but needs additional skills to achieve total suc-

cess. This increases the patient's knowledge of personal capacity. In contrast, the patient has no way of judging competence when engaged in rote exercise.

3. Naturalistic occupations can also divert attention from the pain or discomfort experienced during therapeutic exercise in many clinical conditions. For example, pain management is a major component in the recovery from surgical procedures following hip fracture, and involvement in meaningful, personal occupation while standing can focus attention on other things rather than pain.

4. Skills gained in naturalistic occupations are more likely to transfer to the post-discharge environment than are skills gained in rote exercise. For example, simulated practice of homemaking in the rehabilitation facility is more likely to transfer to skills in the home than participation in isolated movement patterns.

5. Naturalistic occupations typically involve minor variations from time to time, both within sessions and across sessions. For example, each dish or eating utensil to be washed provides a somewhat different challenge, and the dishwashing situation naturally varies from day to day depending on multiple factors. In contrast, exercise alone provides little variation from moment to moment and from session to session. The ability to cope with minor variations may increase the patient's general sense of adaptability to new challenges.

6. The minor variations that are typical of naturalistic occupations (as in # 5 above) may also lead to needed cognitive and sensorimotor skills. Variations are necessary both in the development of cognitive processing strategies and in the learning of advanced motor skills.

7. Rote exercise equipment tends to isolate movement across a single joint with minimal degrees of freedom whereas naturalistic occupations tend to involve several muscle groups and multiple degrees of freedom. For example, most of the muscle groups of the body are involved in using a heavy watering can to water plants. Hence, naturalistic occupations promote coordination of muscles, rather than isolation.

8. Naturalistic occupations tend to provide simultaneous challenges to the sensorimotor, cognitive, and psychosocial abilities of the patient. For example, food preparation can simultaneously challenge fine motor skills, gait and standing balance, communication, problem-solving, coping abilities, and social participation

as a peer. The patient recovering from a hip fracture frequently has multiple impairments and disabilities (the person must not be thought of reductionistically as a "hip").

9. Involvement in naturalistic occupations helps the patient anticipate the future, post-discharge environment. For example, a trip to a shopping mall can encourage the patient to make realistic plans for how this can be accomplished in the future. The patient can become a planner of a personal destiny.

10. Involvement in naturalistic occupations involves the setting of real-life goals. Wanting to provide naturalistic occupational forms, the therapist repeatedly asks the patient to take charge of his/her own rehabilitation. The very act of setting goals can be conceptualized as therapeutic in and of itself.

There also may be disadvantages to the occupationally embedded approach. Sometimes, the distraction of attention that frequently accompanies occupation might lead to the patient's forgetting appropriate post-surgical precautions. Indeed, high levels of motivation could lead the patient to overdo exercise, with negative and sometimes serious consequences, as with the patient who has strict cardiac precautions. A third problem is that naturalistic occupations are not as easy to grade as are exercises on most machines, which provide many different levels of exertion. Finally, the case can be made that specialized therapy equipment is indeed meaningful to some people. In an era in which "working out" has become commonplace for both genders, exercise equipment has become a naturalistic occupational form for many people.

Research in Support of Occupationally Embedded Movement

For over 60 years of occupational therapy's history, no experimental research addressed the relative advantages and disadvantages of occupationally embedded movement and rote exercise. However, in the past 16 years considerable research has addressed this issue. Lin, Wu, Tickle-Degnen, and Coster (1997) conducted a meta-analysis on 17 research studies comparing the effects of occupationally embedded movement and rote exercise. They found effect sizes ranging from -0.07 to 0.92, with a mean effect size of 0.50 in favor of naturalistic occupations. They concluded that their findings "support the concept that naturalistic occupations involving objects may serve as effective means to promote motor performance" (p. 40). Thomas and Nelson (2000) reviewed and analyzed 36 published studies in this topic area (these are cited in the Reference list). Several researchers have contrasted occupationally enhanced forms (including imagery-based forms) and rote exercise in terms of exercise repetitions (e.g., DeKuiper, Nelson, & White, 1993; Hsieh, Nelson, Smith, & Peterson, 1996). Other studies have investigated the amount or range of motion elicited by contrasting occupational forms. Most of these studies have found that occupationally enhanced forms have resulted in more or further movement of designated body parts than rote exercise-based forms (e.g., Nelson, Konosky et al., 1996; Sakemiller & Nelson, 1998). Yet other studies have shown that enhancing occupational forms resulted in greater duration of pain tolerance (Heck, 1988), greater accuracy of drawing (Licht & Nelson, 1990), greater duration of standing tolerance (Hoppes, 1997), greater subjective preference for occupationally embedded exercise (Zimmerer-Branum & Nelson, 1995), and greater accuracy in tracing a maze while using an upper extremity prosthesis (Yuen, Nelson, Peterson, & Dickinson, 1994). Research has been less definitive when investigating physiological responses to contrasting occupational forms in terms of heart rate and blood pressure changes, or psychological response in terms of affective meaning elicited (e.g., Bloch, Nelson, & Smith, 1989).

A recent application of technology designed to quantify aspects of movement has allowed researchers to look not only at the product of movement (e.g., number of repetitions, pain tolerance, degrees of movement, accuracy of drawing) but also at the process of moving. Motion analysis technology permits the investigation of qualities of movement such as movement units (smoothness), movement time (speed), displacement (directness), peak velocity during movement, and the percentage of reach at which peak velocity occurs. Occupational therapy researchers have used this technology to test whether the reaching dynamics during an occupationally embedded movement are different from those elicited by a matched rote exercise or imagery-based movement. Researchers have found that occupationally embedded movement results in a better quality of reach than when engaged in an imagery or rote exercise occupational form. Subjects have included children with cerebral palsy (Beauregard, Thomas, & Nelson, 1998), adults with and without multiple sclerosis (Mathiowetz & Wade, 1995), and female college age students (Hall & Nelson, 1998; Wu, Trombly, & Lin, 1994). The results support the idea that rote exercise is qualitatively different from occupationally embedded movement.

COMMUNICATION, COOPERATION, AND TEAMWORK

Communication for the Sake of the Patient

Physical therapy and occupational therapy are distinct, autonomous professions. It is understandable that each professional group has its own traditions and outlooks. Indeed, the argument can be made that a necessary prerequisite for the integrity of any true profession is a unique philosophy that is distinct from that of any other profession. The two perspectives presented in this paper reflect the respective worldviews of the two professions and mega-trends within those professions. Different terminologies are used, for example. It is not expected that physical therapists use specialized occupational terminology, or vice versa.

Still, physical therapists and occupational therapists must communicate clearly with each other, because they frequently work in teams with the same patients and with other team-members who rely on them. Our recommendation is that physical therapists and occupational therapists work harder at communicating with each other, for the benefit of their patients. For example, it is appropriate and perhaps even necessary for the occupational therapist to be fluent in occupational terminology, because occupation is the core of the profession. But it is also important that the occupational therapist be able to translate specialized terminology into language that team-members, patients, and others will readily understand. Hopefully, papers such as this one will enhance communication by explaining the histories, shifts, and trends of the two professions.

Overlap and Specialization in Roles of Physical Therapists and Occupational Therapists

Members of both professions should acknowledge that both physical therapy and occupational therapy have legitimate roles in the restoration of movement. The physical therapist focuses on human movement as an integral part of everyday life. The occupational therapist focuses on everyday occupations, which consist of human movement. Reductionism, the tendency to focus on a component of the person without consideration of the whole complexity of the person, must be avoided by both professions. The physical therapist would be reductionistic to ignore the tasks of daily life that depend on and challenge movement abilities. And the occupational therapist would be reductionistic to ignore the movement components upon which occupation depends. The foci of the two professions are different, but overlapping concerns are inevitable in patients with movement disorders. For example, the physical therapist has a natural interest in gait, standing tolerance, and dynamic balance for the patient who has had a hip fracture and who is post-status hip surgery. If the best place to observe and treat these abilities is in the context of the patient's cooking a light meal in a kitchen, the physical therapist might well employ this site as a part of best practice for the patient. In parallel fashion, best practice in occupational therapy might also involve a light meal, a kitchen setting, and observations relating to gait, standing tolerance, and dynamic standing balance. We are not saying that physical therapy clinical reasoning and occupational therapy clinical reasoning are exactly the same; we are saying that there is much potential overlap.

How should this overlap be resolved? The rule we suggest is that the best interests of the patient should be the foundation for all decisions relating to specialization and overlap of function between physical therapists and occupational therapists. "Turf wars" involving unresolved decisions concerning division of labor are unacceptable, because they inevitably lead to duplication of services. In turn, duplication of services (e.g., both professions repeatedly conducting range of motion and strength tests, without communication) frequently is accompanied by a failure to provide the full range of services that is desirable and otherwise possible (e.g., a home assessment). Usually, it is a challenge to meet the full rehabilitation needs of a patient, even without unnecessary duplication. The overall motivation of the patient declines if asked naively in the afternoon to do the same thing done all morning with someone else; excessive fatigue of specific muscle groups is another undesirable consequence of failure of interdisciplinary communication. Therapist insensitivity to the discomfort and pain that necessarily accompany recovery from disorders such as hip fracture is unacceptable. Patients have a right to know that therapists communicate successfully with each other, toward the goal of a coherent, integrated plan of intervention.

We recommend that clear guidelines for disciplinary specialization and interdisciplinary teamwork be developed at a local level within each facility. These guidelines should structure decision-making within each rehabilitation team meeting or care plan conference. In addition, one-to-one communication between the physical therapy practitioner and the occupational therapy practitioner is regularly needed to achieve an intervention plan with goals and methods oriented to the unique needs of the individual patient. This type of communication is facilitated when rehabilitation administrators structure teams where individual therapists and therapy assistants work regularly together, as opposed to randomly changing teams.

A special problem of interdisciplinary teams occurs in times of personnel change and the presence of new students. For example, the advent at a facility of a new physical therapist committed to a functional approach and/or to task-oriented exercise might require the restructuring of the guidelines for disciplinary specialization and interdisciplinary teamwork. It is important that decision-making be done in a clear and timely way. For example, observation of lower extremity dressing by the patient with hip fracture could provide the physical therapist with an excellent context for analyzing and enhancing lower extremity range of motion and strength. However, if the facility's tradition called for this to be done by the occupational therapist, unnecessary duplication of services and problems of teamwork predictably develop unless clear communication and decision-making precedes the change in the facility's traditions. Of course, the same principle applies to changes initiated by occupational therapy staff. Flexibility in the facility's traditions and guidelines is necessary to accommodate new ideas about the restoration of movement and new personnel with special training and competencies. Shifts in both professions can be anticipated, especially given the increased emphasis on evidence-based research. Yet the fundamental philosophies, histories, and outlooks of the two professions will remain distinct, as is appropriate for separate professions.

Although we recommend that interdisciplinary guidelines for specialization and teamwork are best made at the facility level, the distinct philosophies, histories, and outlooks of each professional group should guide these decisions. Rehabilitation for persons with hip fracture provides an example. Current practice guidelines (e.g., Russell & Palmieri, 1996) call for rote exercises such as the prone hip extensions, supine straight leg raising, isometric setting exercises of the gluteus maximus, and side-lying hip abduction exercises. These essential exercises are within the physical therapy tradition. To some extent, imagery can often provide motivation while structuring the quality of movement. While performing the traditional hip extension exercise, the individual might be encouraged to imagine swimming or shaking dirt from the bottom of a shoe. Although the protocols for these exercises are quite specific, it is also within the physical therapy tradition to individualize methods of eliciting movement, with consideration of cognitive, communicative, and psychosocial factors.

The guidelines of Russell and Palmieri (1996) for hip fracture also call for self-care training. We recommend that self-care training be initiated by the occupational therapist as soon as possible (we do not think that a period of rote exercise must precede involvement in everyday occupations). In the context of morning hygiene and dressing, the occupational therapist naturally addresses patterns of movement at the hip as well as other muscle regions that may have been affected by deconditioning or co-morbidities. The occupational therapist should also take a leadership role in assessing the patient's occupational goals after rehabilitation. The patient's unique goals and anticipated post-discharge situation should structure the goals and methods of both the physical therapist and the occupational therapist. Rote exercises can be especially effective in developing raw muscle strength and range of motion, but treatment of the patient's isolated deficiencies must always be accompanied by consideration of what the individual patient wants to do and needs to do in life. This principle also applies to gait and balance training. While performing marching in place, for instance, the individual could imagine walking through a favorite grocery store or mall. During this same phase of therapy, the individual could also take daily walks in a preferred setting, could push a grocery cart in place of a walker, or could carry a small sack of groceries in place of dumbbells. The same principle applies to the development of the upper extremities, trunk, and back, all important for the person who has experienced a hip fracture secondary to falling.

CONCLUSION

Properly managed, the overlap between physical therapy and occupational therapy in the restoration of movement becomes an advantage in rehabilitation, not a disadvantage. Both disciplines consider the patient holistically. However, the foci of the two disciplines vary because of the different traditions and outlooks of the two professions. Indeed, in therapeutic interventions with some populations (e.g., those only requiring physical modalities, or those only with cognitive or psychosocial deficits), there may be little overlap between physical therapy and occupational therapy (and perhaps overlap with other disciplines). In the case of patients with movement disorders, the special physical therapy focus is on the musculoskeletal components of human movement, while never forgetting that these movements must be understood as an integral part of everyday life. The special occupational therapy focus is on the occupational configuration of the person, while never forgetting the critical role of movement in daily occupations. With mutual respect, administrative support, and good communication, these complementary perspectives can be put to maximum service in the rehabilitation of persons with movement impairments.

REFERENCES

Ades, P. A., Ballor, D. L., Ashikaga, T., Utton, J. L., & Nair, K. S. (1996). Weight training improves walking endurance in healthy elderly persons. *Annals of Internal Medicine, 124* (6), 568-572.

Anderson, M. A., Gieck, J. H., Perrin, D., Weltman, A., Rutt, R., & Denegar, C. (1991). The relationships among isometric, isotonic, and isokinetic concentric and eccentric quadriceps and hamstring force and three components of athletic performance. *Journal of Orthopaedic and Sports Physical Therapy, 14,* 114-120.

Augustsson, J., Esko, A., Thomee, R., & Svantsesson, U. (1998). Weight training of the thigh muscles using closed vs. open kinetic chain exercises: A comparison of performance enhancement. *Journal of Orthopaedic and Sports Physical Therapy, 27,* 3-8.

Bakshi, R., Bhambhani, Y., & Madill, H. (1991). The effects of task preference on performance during purposeful and nonpurposeful activities. *American Journal of Occupational Therapy, 45* (10), 912-916.

Baldwin, B. T. (1919). *Occupational therapy applied to restoration of movement.* Washington, DC: Commanding Officer and Surgeon General of the Army, Walter Reed General Hospital.

Beauregard, R., Thomas, J. J., & Nelson, D. L. (1998). Quality of reach during a game and during a rote movement in children with cerebral palsy. *Physical & Occupational Therapy in Pediatrics, 18* (3/4), 67-84.

Blackburn, J. R., & Morrissey, M. C. (1998). The relationship between open and closed kinetic chain strength of the lower limb and jumping performance. *Journal of Orthopaedic and Sports Physical Therapy, 27,* 430-435.

Bloch, M. W., Smith, D. A., & Nelson, D. L. (1989). Heart rate, activity and affect in added-purpose versus single-purpose jumping activities. *American Journal of Occupational Therapy, 43* (1), 25-30.

Brotzman, S. B., & Head, P. (1996). The knee. In S. B. Brotzman (Ed.), *Clinical Orthopaedic Rehabilititation* (pp. 183-244). St. Louis, MO: Mosby

Cipriani, D. & Vermillion, R. (1995). Knee rehabilitation: The challenge of function. *Training and Conditioning, 5* (5), 15-24.

Cohn, E. (1908). The systematic occupation and entertainment of the insane in public institutions. *Journal of the American Medical Association, 50,* 1249-1251.

Cress, M. E., Buchner, D. M., Questad, K. A., Esselman, P. C., deLateur, B. J., & Schwartz, R. S. (1999). Exercise: Effects on physical functional performance in independent older adults. *Journal of Gerontology: Medical Sciences, 54A* (5), M242-M248.

DeKuiper, W. P., Nelson, D. L., & White, B. E. (1993). Materials-based occupation versus imagery-based occupation versus rote exercise: A replication and extension. *Occupational Therapy Journal of Research, 13* (3), 183-197.

Dunton, W. R., Jr. (1928). *Prescribing occupational therapy.* Springfield, IL: Charles C. Thomas.

Duscha, B., Cipriani, D., & Roberts, C. (1999). A review of open vs. closed kinetic chain exercise for lower extremity rehabilitation. *Clinical Exercise Physiology, 1* (2), 57-63.

Fitzgerald, G. K. (1997). Open versus closed kinetic chain exercises: Issues in rehabilitation after anterior cruciate ligament reconstructive surgery. *Physical Therapy, 77,* 1747-1754.

Fu, F., Woo, S., & Irrgang, J. (1992). Current concepts for rehabilitation following anterior cruciate ligament reconstruction. *Journal of Orthopaedic and Sports Physical Therapy, 15,* 270-278.

Gray, G. W. (1993). *Chain reaction: Successful strategies for closed chain and open chain testing and rehabilitation.* Adrian, MI: Wynn Marketing, Inc.

Greenberger, H. B., & Paterno, M. V. (1995). Relationship of knee extensor strength and hopping test performance in the assessment of lower extremity function. *Journal of Sports Physical Therapy, 22,* 202-206.

Hall, B. A., & Nelson, D. L. (1998). The effect of materials on performance: A kinematic analysis of eating. *Scandinavian Journal of Occupational Therapy, 5,* 69-81.

Heck, S. A. (1988). The effect of purposeful activity on pain tolerance. *American Journal of Occupational Therapy, 42,* 577-581.

Hoppes, S. (1997). Can play increase standing tolerance? A pilot-study. *Physical & Occupational Therapy in Geriatrics, 15* (1), 65-73.

Hsieh, C. L., Nelson, D. L., Smith, D. A., & Peterson, C. Q. (1996). A comparison of performance in added-purpose occupations and rote exercise for dynamic standing balance in persons with hemiplegia. *American Journal of Occupational Therapy, 50* (1), 10-16.

Jenkins, W., Bronner, S., & Mangine, R. (1997). Functional evaluation and rehabilitation of the lower extremity. In B. Brownstein & S. Bronner (Eds.), *Functional movement in orthopaedic and sports physical therapy: Evaluation, treatment, and outcomes* (pp. 191-230). New York: Churchill Livingstone.

Johnson, S.C. (1920). Instruction in handicrafts and design for hospital patients. *The Modern Hospital, 15,* 1-4.

Judge, J. O., Underwood, M., & Gennosa, T. (1993). Exercise to improve gait velocity in older persons. *Archives of Physical Medicine and Rehabilitation, 74,* 400-406.

King, T. I. (1993). Hand strengthening with a computer for purposeful activity. *American Journal of Occupational Therapy, 47* (7), 635-637.

Kircher, M. A. (1984). Motivation as a factor of perceived exertion in purposeful versus non-purposeful activity. *American Journal of Occupational Therapy, 38* (3), 165-170.

Lang, E. M., Nelson, D. L., & Bush, M. A. (1992). Comparison of performance in materials-based occupation, imagery-based occupation, and rote exercise in nursing home residents. *American Journal of Occupational Therapy, 46* (7), 607-611.

Lentell, G., Baas, B., Lopez, D., McGuire, L., Sarrels, M., & Snyder, P. (1995). The contribution of proprioceptive deficits, muscle function, and anatomic laxity to functional instability of the ankle. *Journal of Orthopaedic and Sports Physical Therapy, 21*, 206-215.

Licht, B. C., & Nelson, D. L. (1990). Adding meaning to a design copy task through representational stimuli. *American Journal of Occupational Therapy, 44* (5), 408-413.

Lin, K., Wu, C., Tickle-Degnen, L., & Coster, W. (1997). Enhancing occupational performance through occupationally embedded exercise: A meta-analytic review. *Occupational Therapy Journal of Research, 17* (1), 25-47.

Mathiowetz, V., & Wade, M. G. (1995). Task constraints and functional motor performance of individuals with and without multiple sclerosis. *Ecological Psychology, 7* (2), 99-123.

Maurer, T. L., Smith, D. A., & Armetta, C. L. (1989). Single purpose vs. added purpose activity: Performance comparisons with chronic schizophrenics. *Occupational Therapy in Mental Health, 9* (3), 9-20.

Miller, L., & Nelson, D. L. (1987). Dual-purpose activity versus single-purpose activity in terms of duration on task, exertion level, and affect. *Occupational Therapy in Mental Health, 7* (1), 55-67.

Morrissey, M. C., Harman, E. A., & Johnson, M. J. (1995). Resistance training modes: Specificity and effectiveness. *Medicine and Science in Sports and Exercise, 27*, 648-660.

Morton, G. G., Barnett, D. W., & Hale, L. S. (1992). A comparison of performance measures of an added-purpose task versus a single purpose task for upper extremities. *American Journal of Occupational Therapy, 46* (2), 128-133.

Moyer, J. A., & Nelson, D. L. (1998). Replication and resynthesis of an occupationally embedded exercise with adult rehabilitation patients. *Israel Journal of Occupational Therapy, 7* (3), E57-E75.

Mullins, C. S., Nelson, D. L., & Smith, D. A. (1987). Exercise through dual-purpose activity in the institutionalized elderly. *Physical & Occupational Therapy in Geriatrics, 5* (3), 29-39.

Nelson, D. L. (1988). Occupation: Form and performance. *American Journal of Occupational Therapy, 42* (10), 633-641.

Nelson, D. L. (1994). Form and function. In C. B. Royeen (Ed.), *AOTA self-study series: The practice of the future: Putting occupation back into therapy* (lesson 2), Bethesda, MD: American Occupational Therapy Association.

Nelson, D. L., Konosky, K., Fleharty, K., Webb, R., Newer, K., Hazboun, V. P., Fontaine, C., & Licht, B. (1996). The effects of an occupationally embedded exercise on bilaterally assisted supination in persons with hemiplegia. *American Journal of Occupational Therapy, 50*, 639-646.

Nelson, D. L., & Peterson, C. Q. (1989). Enhancing therapeutic exercise through purposeful activity: A theoretical analysis. *Topics in Geriatric Rehabilitation, 4*, 12-22.

Paul, S., & Ramsey, D. (1998). The effects of electronic music-making as a therapeutic activity for improving active range of motion. *Occupational Therapy International, 5* (33), 223-237.

Riccio, C. M., Nelson, D. L., & Bush, M. A. (1990). Adding purpose to the repetitive exercise of elderly women through imagery. *American Journal of Occupational Therapy, 44* (8), 714-719.

Rice, M. S. (1998). Purposefulness and cross transfer in a forearm supination and pronation task. *Scandinavian Journal of Occupational Therapy, 5* (1), 31-37.

Ross, L. M., & Nelson, D. L. (2000). Comparing materials-based occupation, imagery-based occupation, and rote movement through kinematic analysis of reach. *Occupational Therapy Journal of Research, 20,* 45-60.

Rozzi, S. L., Lephart, S. M., Sterner, R., & Kuligowski, L. (1999). Balance training for persons with functionally unstable ankles. *Journal of Orthopaedic and Sports Physical Therapy, 29* (8), 478-486.

Russell, T. A., & Palmieri, A. K. (1996). Fractures of the pelvis, acetabulum, and lower extremity. In S.B. Brotzman (Ed.), *Clinical Orthopaedic Rehabilititation* (pp. 143-182) St. Louis, MO: Mosby.

Sakemiller, L. M., & Nelson, D. L. (1998). Eliciting functional extension in prone through the use of a game. *American Journal of Occupational Therapy, 52* (2), 150-157.

Schmidt, C. L., & Nelson, D. L. (1996). A comparison of three occupational forms in rehabilitation inpatients receiving upper extremity strengthening. *Occupational Therapy Journal of Research, 16,* 200-215.

Sietsema, J. M., Nelson, D. L., Mulder, R. M., Mervau-Scheidel, D., & White, B. E. (1993). The use of a game to promote arm reach in persons with traumatic brain injury. *American Journal of Occupational Therapy, 47* (1), 19-24.

Steinbeck, T. M. (1986). Purposeful activity and performance. *American Journal of Occupational Therapy, 40* (8), 529-534.

Thibodeaux, C. S., & Ludwig, F. M. (1988). Intrinsic motivation in product oriented and non-product oriented activities. *American Journal of Occupational Therapy, 42* (3), 169-175.

Thomas, J. J. (1996). Materials-based, imagery-based, and rote exercise occupational forms: Effect on repetitions, heart rate, duration of performance, and self-perceived rest period in well elderly women. *American Journal of Occupational Therapy, 50* (10), 783-789.

Thomas, J. J., & Nelson, D. L. (2000). Moving toward a scientific base for one of the oldest and most important ideas in the profession of occupational therapy. In J. Hinojosa & M. L. Blount (Eds.), *The texture of life: Purposeful activities in occupational therapy* (pp. 394-419). Bethesda, MD: American Occupational Therapy Association.

Thomas, J. J., Vander Wyk, S. A., & Boyer, J. (1999). Contrasting occupational forms: Effects on performance and affect in patients undergoing phase II cardiac rehabilitation. *Occupational Therapy Journal of Research, 19,* 187-202.

van der Weel, F. R., van der Meer, A. L. H., & Lee, D. N. (1991). Effect of task on movement control in cerebral palsy: Implications for assessment and therapy. *Developmental Medicine and Child Neurology, 33,* 419-426.

Wagner, M. R., Krauss, A., & Horowitz, B. (1995). Occupationally embedded exercise, rote exercise, and the presence of another person in the exercise context. *The Israel Journal of Occupational Therapy, 4* (4), E87-E101.

Worrell, T. W., Borchert, B., Erner, K., Fritz, J., & Leerar, P. (1993). Effect of a lateral step-up exercise protocol on quadriceps and lower extremity performance. *Journal of Orthopaedic and Sports Physical Therapy, 18,* 646-653.

Wu, C., Trombly, C. A., & Lin, K. (1994). The relationship between occupational form and occupational performance: A kinematic perspective. *American Journal of Occupational Therapy, 48* (8), 679-687.

Yack, H. J., Collins, C. E., & Whieldon, T. J. (1993). Comparison of closed and open kinetic chain exercise in the anterior cruciate ligament-deficient knee. *American Journal of Sports Medicine, 21,* 49-54.

Yoder, R. M., Nelson, D. L., & Smith, D. A. (1989). Added-purpose versus rote exercise in female nursing home residents. *American Journal of Occupational Therapy, 43* (9), 581-586.

Yuen, H. K., Nelson, D. L., Peterson, C. Q., & Dickenson, A. (1994). Prosthesis training as a context for studying occupational forms and motoric adaptation. *American Journal of Occupational Therapy, 48* (1), 55-61.

Zimmerer-Branum, S., & Nelson, D. L. (1995). Occupationally embedded exercise versus rote exercise: A choice between forms by elderly nursing home residents. *American Journal of Occupational Therapy, 49,* 394-402.

Dementia, Nutrition, and Self-Feeding: A Systematic Review of the Literature

Cathy D. Dolhi, MS, OTR/L
Joan C. Rogers, PhD, OTR/L, FAOTA

SUMMARY. The outcomes of feeding training are typically evaluated in terms of feeding skills and swallowing abilities rather than the ultimate goal of feeding, namely, adequate nutritional status. To increase occupational therapy practitioners' awareness of nutritional status as an outcome of feeding training, a systematic review of the research literature was conducted to examine the relationship between nutritional status and self-feeding skills in people with dementia. Studies were evaluated by the strength of their evidence and analyzed to determine the relationships among dementia, nutritional status, and the ability to feed one's self. Results revealed that although nutritional status in people with dementia is variable, there is a tendency for lower body weight, lower measures of body composition, and lower body mass indexes in persons with dementia compared to those with no cognitive impairment. Individuals who feed themselves tend to weigh more compared

Cathy D. Dolhi is Assistant Professor, Occupational Therapy Department, Chatham College, Pittsburgh, PA 15232.

Joan C. Rogers is Professor and Chair, Occupational Therapy Department, University of Pittsburgh, Pittsburgh, PA 15260.

The authors thank Evelyn C. Granieri, MD, and Margo B. Holm, PhD, OTR/L, FAOTA, ABDA, for reviewing and contributing to drafts of this work.

Address correspondence to: Cathy D. Dolhi, MS, OTR/L, Occupational Therapy Department, Chatham College, Woodland Road, Pittsburgh, PA 15232.

[Haworth co-indexing entry note]: "Dementia, Nutrition, and Self-Feeding: A Systematic Review of the Literature." Dolhi, Cathy D., and Joan C. Rogers. Co-published simultaneously in *Occupational Therapy in Health Care* (The Haworth Press, Inc.) Vol. 15, No. 3/4, 2001, pp. 59-87; and: *Interprofessional Collaboration in Occupational Therapy* (ed: Stanley Paul, and Cindee Q. Peterson) The Haworth Press, Inc., 2001, pp. 59-87. Single or multiple copies of this article are available for a fee from The Haworth Document Delivery Service [1-800-HAWORTH, 9:00 a.m. - 5:00 p.m. (EST). E-mail address: getinfo@haworthpressinc.com].

59

to those who need assistance for feeding. There is also evidence to support that as feeding status improves or declines, body weight similarly increases or decreases. *[Article copies available for a fee from The Haworth Document Delivery Service: 1-800-HAWORTH. E-mail address: <getinfo@ haworthpressinc.com> Website: <http://www.HaworthPress.com> © 2001 by The Haworth Press, Inc. All rights reserved.]*

KEYWORDS. Alzheimer's disease, undernutrition, self-feeding skills, review article

INTRODUCTION

Dementia is highly prevalent in the United States with 4 million Americans being affected by Alzheimer's disease (AD) alone (National Institute on Aging, 1999). Dementias of the chronic, progressive type impair cognitive capabilities and eventually alter the ability to perform even basic tasks. The inability to remember, plan and execute movement, and express one's needs negatively affects participation in activities that were once familiar, routine, and completed nearly at a subconscious level. Once independent and productive members of their community, people with dementia are confronted with difficulty performing tasks as fundamental as bathing, dressing, toileting, and eating. As a result, many rely on family members or paid caregivers to assist them in their daily self-care routines.

Research suggests that weight loss and malnutrition are common in people with dementia (Watson, 1997). Some researchers propose that a decline in body weight and a propensity for malnutrition occur as a result of the pathophysiology of dementia (Barrett-Connor, Edelstein, Corey-Bloom, & Wiederholt, 1996; Reyes-Ortega et al., 1997; White, Pieper, & Schmader, 1998; White, Pieper, Schmader, & Fillenbaum, 1996). Others suggest that these conditions are directly related to a decreased ability to shop for, prepare, and/or eat food as well as feed one's self (Berkhout, Cools, & van Houwelingen, 1998; Berlinger & Potter, 1991; Du, DiLuca, & Growdon, 1993; Wang, Fukagawa, Hossain, & Ooi, 1997). Understanding the evidence that supports these perspectives is important to occupational therapy practitioners, who frequently treat people with performance deficits in feeding and eating secondary to dementia. According to the first hypothesis, feeding interventions would have little influence on improving nutritional status because weight loss and malnutrition are indigenous to dementia. According to the second hypothesis, feeding interventions could potentially prevent or reverse malnutrition.

If the evidence supporting the relationship between feeding abilities and nutritional status is substantive, occupational therapy practitioners may need to broaden their frame of reference for eating and feeding interventions. Currently, intervention focuses on the motor, cognitive, and psychosocial components of eating and feeding with less attention given to the desired outcome of maintaining good nutritional status or improving compromised nutritional status. Attention is directed toward selecting and using appropriate eating utensils, bringing food or drink to the mouth, sucking and swallowing, making food preferences known to caregivers, and being socially appropriate (American Occupational Therapy Association, 2000; Holm, Rogers, & James, 1998; Trombly, 1995). The ability to self-feed and eat takes precedence over the desired outcome of these tasks, adequate nutritional intake. Thus, intervention may result in increased independence in feeding but decreased nutritional intake, for example, when clients eat less food or less nutritious food because they tire easily or eat dessert rather than the peas and carrots.

To assist practitioners to understand the relationship between dementia, nutrition, and feeding ability, a systematic literature review was conducted to answer two research questions:

1. What is the relationship between dementia and nutritional status, as measured by biochemical indices, anthropometric measures, weight loss, and dietary intake?
2. What is the relationship between nutritional status and self-feeding status in people with dementia?

METHOD

To examine the relationship between dementia, nutritional status, and feeding, the research literature was searched from 1980 through 1999. This was accomplished using the Cumulative Index of Nursing and Allied Health Literature (CINAHL) and Medline using the search terms dementia, nutrition, malnutrition, undernutrition, and feeding. To be included in the review, articles had to be written in English and examine nutrition in relation to dementia, or, feeding status of people with dementia in relation to nutritional status. Case reports and review articles that were not systematic were excluded. The search strategy yielded 19 studies: three cross sectional, six essentially cross sectional with longitudinal components for weight or mortality, nine longitudinal, and one intervention. Research articles were ranked by the strength of evidence using the hierarchy proposed by Moore, McQuay and Gray (1995) with Level I indicating the strongest evidence and Level V the weakest evidence. Level 1 includes evidence from at least one systematic literature review of multiple well-designed randomized controlled clinical trials; Level II includes evidence from at least one well-designed randomized controlled trial; Level III includes evidence from non-randomized clinical trials, and studies involving pretests and post-tests of a single group, a cohort, time series, or case-controls; Level IV includes evidence from non-experimental studies enrolling subjects from more than one center or group of investigators; and Level V includes expert opinion based on clinical evidence, descriptive studies and expert panels. On Tables 1 through 3, studies are listed first by level of evidence and then alphabetically within each level.

NUTRITIONAL STATUS AND DEMENTIA

Malnutrition, which includes overnutrition and undernutrition, is a compromised state of nutrition in which the body cells receive inappropriate amounts of one or more nutrients (Lutz & Przytulski, 1997). Undernutrition is considered in this review because of its prevalence in people with dementia. A brief description of the clinical manifestations of undernutrition and the parameters commonly used to assess it is provided to familiarize occupational therapy practitioners with the terms and concepts related to nutrition. The significance of the parameters as they relate to well nourished and malnourished states is presented.

Undernutrition affects 10% to 20% of elders who live in the community and up to 60% of those in long-term and acute care facilities (Clarke, Wahlqvist, & Strauss, 1998). Muscle wasting and weakness, increased risk of infection, increased potential for skin breakdown, high frequency of hospitalizations, and nursing home placement are commonly associated with undernutrition (Chapman & Nelson, 1994; Morley, 1996; Sandman, Adolfsson, Nygren, Hallmans, & Winblad, 1987). Although the consequences of undernutrition are universal, there is little consensus about the specific criteria for defining it (Kerstetter, Holthausen, & Fitz, 1992). Despite the lack of a "gold standard" (Bartlett, 1998; Silver, Morley, Strome, Jones, & Vicker, 1988; Thomas, Verdery, Gardner, Kant, & Lindsay, 1991), biochemical indices,

TABLE 1. Studies Using Biochemical and Anthropometric Indicators of Nutritional Status

Study	Subject characteristics	Biochemical parameters	Body composition	Body weight & BMI
Barrett-Connor et al. (1996) Longitudinal design (20 years) Level III	<u>With dementia</u> • **Community based** • 24 women / 77.2 ± 4.4 years • 36 men / 77.4 ± 4.2 years • MMSE 24.2 ± 3.5 women; 21.6 ± 5.6 men <u>Without dementia</u> • **Community based** • 141 women / 71.8 ± 6.7 years • 98 men / 71.3 ± 7.3 years • MMSE scores not reported			Weight loss occurred prior to the dementia diagnosis. Weight loss significant over 3 measurement periods, spanning 20 years, in Ss eventually diagnosed with possible or probable AD. Cognitively intact Ss had no significant weight change.
Berlinger & Potter (1991) Cross-sectional design Level III	<u>With dementia</u> • **Community based** • Group II–Probable/possible AD 79 women / 42 men Sample age 79 ± 7 years MMSE 16 ± 6 • Group III–Other dementia 49 women / 16 men Sample age 79 ± 8 years MMSE 16 ± 6 <u>Without dementia</u> • **Community based** Group I–Cognitively intact / No depression 47 women / 6 men Sample age 77 ± 7 years MMSE 25 ± 6 • Group IV–Depressed/Mixed with (n = 44) & without dementia (n = 62) 81 women / 26 men Sample age 78 ± 7 years MMSE 22 ± 6	No difference in serum albumin levels among 4 study groups		BMI significantly lower in Ss with dementia (Groups II, III, & IV) than cognitively intact Ss (Group I).

TABLE 1 (continued)

Study	Subject characteristics	Biochemical parameters	Body composition	Body weight & BMI
Burns et al. (1989) Cross-sectional design with longitudinal (6 months) analysis for weight Level III	**With dementia** <u></u> • **Community based** • 23 women / 5 men • Sample age 80.1 ± 7.3 years • MMSE 3.8 ± 7.0 • **Institutionalized** • 16 women / 5 men • Sample age 81.1 ± 5.7 years • MMSE 2.9 ± 5.9 **Without dementia** • **Community based** • 19 women / 10 men • Sample age 80.3 ± 6.2 years • MMSE 30 ± 0.2	No significant difference in serum albumin + 17 other biochemical parameters.	Ss with dementia had smaller mid-arm & arm-muscle circumference & triceps skinfold thickness than Ss without dementia. Differences significant only for institutionalized Ss with dementia.	Institutionalized Ss with dementia weighed significantly less than community based Ss with & without dementia, but all Ss with dementia weighed less than those without dementia. Institutionalized, but not community based, Ss with dementia lost weight over 6 months. BMI in institutionalized Ss with dementia was significantly lower than community based Ss with & without dementia. Difference between the 2 community based groups not significant.
Franklin & Karkeck (1989) Longitudinal design (17-19 months) Level III	**With dementia** • **Institutionalized** • 36 Ss / 85 years **Without dementia** • **Institutionalized** • 31 Ss / 88 years			Ss with AD weighed significantly less than cognitively intact Ss on admission to institution. Both groups lost weight over time but Ss with AD lost significantly more weight.

Study	Subject characteristics	Biochemical parameters	Body composition	Body weight & BMI
Franzoni et al. (1996) Cross-sectional design with longitudinal analysis (28 months) for mortality Level III	**With dementia** **Institutionalized** • 30 women / 3 men • Sample age 85.7 ± 5.7 years • MMSE 11.4 ± 6.1 **Without dementia** **Institutionalized** • 22 women / 3 men • Sample age 84.9 ± 5.7 years • MMSE 25.1 ± 3.7	Tendency for serum albumin + 4 other biochemical parameters to be lower in Ss with dementia. Differences between Ss with and without dementia not significant.	Triceps skinfold thickness significantly smaller in Ss with than without dementia. Mid-arm circumference also smaller for Ss with dementia, but difference not significant.	Ss with dementia weighed less than Ss without dementia, but difference not significant. Ss with dementia had lower BMI than Ss without dementia, but difference not significant.
Singh et al. (1988) Cross-sectional design with longitudinal (retrospective) analysis of body weight Level III	**With dementia** **Institutionalized** • 29 women (AD) / 86.2 ± 6.5 years • 20 women (MID) / 83 ± 6.6 years • Degree of dementia not reported **Without dementia** **Institutionalized** • 25 women / 80.9 ± 6.1 years	No significant differences in serum albumin + 9 other biochemical parameters between Ss with AD, MID & without dementia.	Ss with AD, but not MID, had significantly lower arm-muscle circumference than Ss without dementia. Ss with AD had less fat free mass than Ss with MID and without dementia. Ss with AD & MID had less body fat than Ss without dementia, & Ss with AD had less than Ss with MID.	Ss with AD weighed significantly less than Ss with MID & Ss without dementia. Difference between Ss with MID & Ss without dementia not significant. Ss with AD lost weight in 2 years before onset of cognitive symptoms.
Spindler et al. (1996) Longitudinal design (1 year) Level III	**With dementia** **Institutionalized** • 11 women / 80.6 ± 6.2 years • 6 men / 76.6 ± 7.6 years • Degree of dementia not reported **Without dementia** **Community based** • 14 women / 71.9 ± 7.2 years • 9 men / 72.9 ± 5.9 years	Women with AD had significantly lower serum albumin values compared to cognitively intact women with no significant change over 1 year (Serum protein was also lower and IGF-1 higher). Serum albumin and other levels not significantly different in males.		Ss with AD weighed less than controls, but difference not significant. No change in body weight in either group over 12 months. Women with AD had significantly lower BMI than cognitively intact counterparts. BMI not significantly different among male Ss.

TABLE 1 (continued)

Study	Subject characteristics	Biochemical parameters	Body composition	Body weight & BMI
White et al. (1996) Longitudinal design (1-5 years) Level III	**With dementia** • **CERAD data base** • 185 women / 72.5 ± 8.3 years • 177 men / 70.1 ± 7.2 years • Clinical Dementia Rating Scale • 0.5 = 10; 1 = 208; 2 = 136; 3 = 8 **Without dementia** • **Community based** • 211 women / 68.1 ± 8.0 years • 106 men / 70.9 ± 6.8 years • Clinical Dementia Rating Scale 0 = 317			Nearly twice as many Ss with AD lost clinically significant amounts of weight during the study (average 2.3 years for AD Ss & 2.9 years for controls) compared to cognitively intact Ss. Weight loss increased with greater functional impairment (measured by Blessed Dementia Rating Scale at study initiation).
Winograd et al. (1991) Cross-sectional design Level III	**With dementia** • **Community based** • 12 women / 66 ± 7 years • 23 men / 68 ± 8 years • MMSE 9 ± 6 women; 17 ± 8 men **Without dementia** • **Community based** • 5 women / 74 ± 6 years • 24 men / 67 ± 7 years • MMSE 28 ± 0.6 women; 29 ± 1.0 men	Serum albumin + 6 other biochemical parameters within normal limits for both groups.		No significant difference in percent of ideal body weight between Ss with and without dementia. BMI slightly less in Ss with dementia but difference not significant.
White et al. (1998) Longitudinal design (6 years) Level IV	**With dementia** • **CERAD data base** • 380 women / 72.0 ± 8.0 years • 286 men / 71.0 ± 8.0 years • Clinical Dementia Rating Scale • 0.5 = 4%; 1 = 54%; 2 = 37%; 3 = 5% **Without dementia** • None			Weight loss associated with AD severity & progression during study (mean time 2.3 ± 1.3 years). As disease severity increased, weight loss increased and/or as Ss lost weight, disease progressed.

66

Study	Subject characteristics	Biochemical parameters	Body composition	Body weight & BMI
Reyes-Ortega et al. (1997) Cross-sectional design with longitudinal analysis (6 months) of body weight Level V	With dementia • Hospitalized • 6 women/ 6 men • Sample age 74.5 ± 6.5 years • MMSE 15.6 ± 7.6 Without dementia • None	Serum albumin + 2 other biochemical parameters were normal	Body composition did not correlate with any other variable.	Ss had mean weight loss of 4.25 ± 2.99 pounds within 6 months prior to study. Weight & BMI not correlated with any other variable.
Sandman et al. (1987) Cross-sectional design with longitudinal analysis (1-36 months) of body weight Level V	With dementia • Institutionalized • 10 women / 8 men • Sample age 73.0 ± 7.0 years • Berger Dementia Rating Scale 4.5 ± 0.9 Without dementia • None	Serum albumin + 17 other biochemical parameters were measured. A majority had normal values on 3 indicators of malnutrition: serum albumin (82.4%); serum transferrin (71.6%); pre-albumin (82.4%).	72% had low triceps skinfold thickness & 50% low arm-muscle circumference compared to reference values.	50% low values of reference weight. Ss with AD weighed more on admission & lost significantly more weight than Ss with MID.
Stähelin et al. (1983) Longitudinal design (3 weeks) Level V	With dementia • Institutionalized • 6 women / 85 years • Degree of dementia not reported Without dementia • None	Serum albumin & total serum protein within normal limits.		Ss maintained stable body weights over 3 weeks.

Note: Age expressed as mean ± standard deviation, if reported; AD = Alzheimer's disease; MID = Multi-infarct dementia; MMSE = Mini-Mental State Examination, expressed as mean ± standard deviation, if reported; Ss = Subjects; BMI = Body mass index

TABLE 2. Studies Reporting Dietary Intake as a Measure of Nutrition

Study	Subject characteristics	Intake measurement method	Results
Burns et al. (1989) Cross-sectional design with longitudinal (6 months) analysis for weight Level III	**With dementia** • **Community based** • 23 women / 5 men • Sample age 80.1 ± 7.3 years • MMSE 3.8 ± 7.0 • **Institutionalized** • 16 women / 5 men • Sample age 81.1 ± 5.7 years • MMSE 2.9 ± 5.9 **Without dementia** • **Community based** • 19 women / 10 men • Sample age 80.3 ± 6.2 years • MMSE 30 ± 0.2	Foods weighed on electronic scale before and after consumption (including spilled food as feasible) for 3 days on randomly selected Ss in 3 study groups. Nutrient content calculated using standard tables.	41% of institutionalized Ss & 33% of community based Ss with dementia met or exceeded Recommended Dietary Allowances for caloric intake. 95% of institutionalized Ss & 83% of community based Ss with dementia reached or exceeded Recommended Dietary Allowances for protein intake. Community based Ss without dementia had significantly lower energy and protein intakes than community based and institutionalized Ss with dementia.
Franzoni et al. (1996) Cross-sectional design with longitudinal analysis (28 months) for mortality Level III	**With dementia** • **Institutionalized** • 30 women / 3 men • Sample age 85.7 ± 5.7 years • MMSE 11.4 ± 6.1 • **Without dementia** • **Institutionalized** • 22 women/ 3 men • Sample age 84.9 ± 5.7 years • MMSE 25.1 ± 3.7	Food weighed before and after consumption for 3 days. Nutrient intake calculated.	No significant difference in intake or nutrient value between Ss with and without dementia.

Study	Subject characteristics	Intake measurement method	Results
Spindler et al. (1996) Longitudinal design (1 year) Level III	<u>With dementia</u> • **Institutionalized** • 11 women / 80.6 ± 6.2 years • 6 men / 76.6 ± 7.6 years • Degree of dementia not reported <u>Without dementia</u> • **Community based** • 14 women / 71.9 ± 7.2 years • 9 men / 72.9 ± 5.9 years	Intake measured at baseline, 6 & 12 months. Food weighed before & after consumption for institutionalized Ss for 2 consecutive days × 3 meals. Adjustments for spill-age, food taken from another, etc. Daily intake reported by community based Ss (4 consecutive days). Nutrient value calculated.	Ss with AD consumed significantly more than Ss without dementia.
Winograd et al. (1991) Cross-sectional design Level III	<u>With dementia</u> • **Community based** • 12 women / 66 ± 7 years • 23 men / 68 ± 8 years • MMSE 9 ± 6 women; 17 ± 8 men <u>Without dementia</u> • **Community based** • 5 women / 74 ± 6 years • 24 men / 67 ± 7 years • MMSE 28 ± 0.6 women; 29 ± 1.0 men	Daily intake (for 3 days) self-reported by Ss without dementia. Informant-report for Ss with dementia (3 days). Nutrient intake calculated.	Nutritional intake of Ss with dementia met Recommended Dietary Allowances & did not differ from cognitively intact Ss.
Sandman et al. (1987) Cross-sectional design with longitudinal analysis (1-36 months) of body weight Level V	<u>With dementia</u> • **Institutionalized** • 10 women / 8 men • Sample age 73.7 ± 7.0 years • Berger Dementia Rating Scale 4.5 ± 0.9 <u>Without dementia</u> • None	Food weighed before and after consumption for 5 consecutive days on 2 occasions. Nutrient intake calculated.	No significant intake deficiencies. Intake higher than calculated needs and exceeded Swedish National Food Administration recommendations. Ss with AD (n = 10) had lower intake than Ss with MID (n = 8). Malnourished Ss had higher intake than Ss who were not malnourished.

TABLE 2 (continued)

Study	Subject characteristics	Intake measurement method	Results
Reyes-Ortega et al. (1997) Cross-sectional design with longitudinal analysis (6 months) of body weight Level V	<u>With dementia</u> • **Hospitalized** • 6 women / 6 men • Sample age 74.5 ± 6.5 years • MMSE 15.6 ± 7.6 <u>Without dementia</u> • None	Estimated from 3-day food records	Wide range of caloric intake (1207-2675 Calories/day for mean of 1782 ± 462.6 Calories/day). No correlation with any other variables.
Stähelin et al. (1983) Longitudinal design (3 weeks) Level V	<u>With dementia</u> • **Institutionalized** • 6 women / 85 years • Degree of dementia not reported <u>Without dementia</u> • None	Food weighed before & after consumption for 2 days/week for 3 weeks. Nutrient value calculated.	Intake sufficient & surpassed protein intake recommendations.
Suski & Nielson (1989) Cross-sectional design Level V	<u>With dementia</u> • **Institutionalized** • 19 women / 89 years • "Late stage" dementia <u>Without dementia</u> • None	Estimated by researcher based on visual inspection (3 days). Nutrient value calculated.	Intake deficient without dietary supplements. Supplements provided 29% of calories & 41.5% of protein.

Note: Age expressed as mean ± standard deviation, if reported; AD = Alzheimer's disease; MID = Multi-infarct dementia; MMSE = Mini-Mental State Examination, expressed as mean ± standard deviation, if reported; Ss = Subjects anthropometric measurements, and dietary intake are commonly used to assess nutritional status.

Biochemical Indices

Although no single biochemical indicator is adequate for predicting protein energy malnutrition, serum albumin is the single most commonly recommended measure (Thomas et al., 1991). Its significance is highlighted by its inclusion, along with body weight, in the Omnibus Reconciliation Act (OBRA) of 1987 as an index of nutritional status in long-term care facilities (Thomas, Kamel, & Morley, 1998). Serum albumin measures simple proteins in the system, with levels under 35 grams per liter reflective of undernutrition in the elderly (Clarke et al., 1998; Gilmore, Robinson, Posthauer, & Raymond, 1995). The invasiveness of drawing blood to obtain biochemical levels may make them difficult or undesirable to obtain in some people.

Of the nine studies that used biochemical indices to measure nutritional status (see Table 1), five Level III studies (Berlinger & Potter, 1991; Burns, Marsh, & Bender, 1989; Franzoni, Frisoni, Boffelli, Rozzini, & Trabucchi, 1996; Singh, Mulley, & Losowsky, 1988; Winograd et al., 1991) and two Level V studies (Reyes-Ortega et al., 1997; Stähelin, Hofer, Vogel, Held, & Seiler, 1983) found no significant difference in serum albumin (or in other biochemical measures) in subjects with dementia when compared with control subjects or laboratory norms. However, another Level III study (Spindler, Renvall, Nichols, & Ramsdell, 1996) found significantly lower levels of serum albumin levels in females (n = 11), but not males with dementia, and one Level V study (Sandman et al., 1987) found low serum albumin levels in 17.6% of subjects with dementia. Thus, although the stronger evidence suggests that the serum albumin levels of subjects with and without dementia do not differ, there is suggestive evidence from both Level III and Level V studies that serum albumin levels may be low in some subjects with dementia.

Anthropometric Measures

Anthropometric measures include indicators of body composition, body weight, and height (Mobarhan & Trumbore, 1991). Mid-arm circumference and triceps skinfold thickness are useful measurements of body composition and nutritional status (Brunt, Schafer, & Oakland, 1999; Morley, Thomas, & Kamel, 1998) because half of the body's protein is stored in muscle tissue (Lutz & Przytulski, 1997). Both measurements are taken midway between the acromion and olecranon with a measuring tape or calipers (Singh et al., 1988; Thomas et al., 1991). They may be used together to determine arm-muscle circumference expressed as: *mid-arm circumference (cm)-[0.314 x triceps skinfold (cm)]* which is also a measure of body composition (Moore, 1997; Sandman et al., 1987; Singh et al., 1988). Anthropometric measures can be performed easily on nearly all patients, are particularly suitable for those who cannot be weighed on conventional scales (Nightingale, Walsh, Bullock, & Wicks, 1996), and over time can provide objective data about amounts of subcutaneous fat and muscle mass.

Of the five studies that used body composition measures of nutritional status (Table 1), three Level III studies (Burns et al., 1989; Franzoni et al., 1996; Singh et al., 1988) found lower values in subjects with dementia. Specifically, Burns et al. (1989) reported lower mid-arm and arm-muscle circumference and triceps skinfold thickness measures in all subjects with dementia compared to those without dementia. Significant differences were present in subjects with dementia who were institutionalized but not for subjects with dementia who were living in the community. Similarly, Franzoni et al. (1996) found reduced triceps skinfold thickness in institutionalized subjects with dementia compared to institutionalized subjects without dementia; however mid-arm circumference was not significantly different. Singh et al. (1988) found reduced arm-muscle circumference in institutionalized subjects with AD but not multi-infarct dementia (MID), compared to institutionalized subjects without dementia. One Level V study (Sandman et al., 1987) study reported low arm-muscle circumferential measurements in 50% of subjects and low triceps skinfold thickness in 72%. A second Level V study (Reyes-Ortega et al., 1997) reported no correlation between nutritional status and body composition when looking exclusively at subjects (n = 12) with AD. Hence, the strongest evidence suggests that people with dementia living in institutions may have lower measures of body composition than those without dementia.

Body weight is a non-invasive, objective, low-cost, readily available, and reliable nutritional index (Bartlett, 1998; Gants, 1997; Mobarhan & Trumbore, 1991; Morley et al., 1998; Silver, 1993). Weight loss is so pervasive in people with dementia that it is a diagnostic feature of probable AD, following the exclusion of other potential causes (McKhann et al., 1984). Body weight was examined in 12 studies (Table 1). With the exception of the Winograd et al. study (1991), all Level III studies (Barrett-Connor et al., 1996; Burns et al., 1989; Franklin & Karkeck,

1989; Franzoni et al., 1996; Singh et al., 1988; Spindler et al., 1996; White et al., 1996) compared subjects with and without dementia and reported lower, although not always significantly lower, body weight in subjects with dementia. In addition, the findings of Burns and colleagues were confined to subjects who were institutionalized and did not extend to community-based subjects with dementia. Compared to those without dementia, greater weight loss over 6 months (Burns et al.) to 20 years (Barrett-Connor et al.) was documented in these studies for subjects with dementia, except for Spindler. One Level V study reported weight loss over 6 months in subjects with dementia (Reyes-Ortega et al., 1997) and another study over an average of 25 months (Sandman et al., 1987). The conflicting findings of the third Level V study (Stähelin et al., 1983), which did not detect a change in body weight, may be attributed to the brief study interval, which was only three weeks. Two studies indicate that weight loss may be more problematic for subjects with AD than MID (Sandman et al.; Singh et al.). Of the studies that did not use cognitively intact controls, one Level IV study (White et al., 1998) reported a significant correlation between weight loss and dementia severity. Thus, the evidence supports the tendency for persons with dementia to have lower body weight than those without dementia and to experience greater weight loss over time.

Body mass index (BMI), calculated as: *body weight in kilograms ÷ (height in meters)^2* is a more sensitive anthropometric measure because it considers weight and height simultaneously. Of the six studies that used BMI as an index of nutritional status (Table 2), five were Level III studies (Berlinger & Potter, 1991; Burns et al., 1989; Franzoni et al., 1996; Spindler et al., 1996; Winograd et al., 1991). Although BMI was lower in subjects with dementia, the difference was significant in only three studies (Berlinger & Potter; Burns et al.; Spindler et al.). Further, the findings of Burns et al. and Spindler et al. were confined to institutionalized subjects with dementia and female subjects with dementia, respectively. In the sixth study, Reyes-Ortega et al. (1997) ascertained that BMI failed to correlate with other nutritional indices such as weight loss, resting energy expenditure, and caloric intake. Thus, there is suggestive evidence that subjects with dementia may have lower BMIs than those without dementia.

Dietary Intake

Dietary intake takes into account the amount and type of food ingested. To track dietary intake, reliable subjects or caregivers may complete intake records. Intake may be estimated by visually inspecting the proportion of food eaten (e.g., 1/2, 3/4) or by weighing the food before and after eating and calculating the amount of food eaten. Weighing is more objective and may yield a more accurate estimate (Pierson, 1999; Simmons & Reuben, 2000). Nonetheless, measuring dietary intake in people with dementia by either method is problematic because of the tendency to spill foods, take food from a plate other than one's own, and pocket food in the cheek only to spit it out later. In addition to the amount of food eaten, its caloric and/or nutritional value is typically calculated either by estimation or commercially available conversion programs.

Eight studies used dietary intake as a measure of nutrition in people with dementia (Table 2). Regardless of the recording method–weighing or self-report, caregiver-report, or researcher-report–only Suski and Nielsen (1989) reported that intake was inadequate for meeting the recommended daily allowances for various vitamins and nutrients. Thus the evidence supporting adequate intake by subjects with dementia comes from four Level III studies (Burns et al., 1989; Franzoni et al., 1996; Spindler et al., 1996; Winograd et al., 1991) and three Level V studies (Reyes-Ortega et al., 1997; Sandman et al., 1987; Stähelin et al., 1983) while that for inadequate intake is gleaned from a Level V study (Suski & Nielsen).

NUTRITIONAL STATUS AND SELF-FEEDING

Self-feeding, the ability to use one's hands to transport food to the mouth, was frequently mentioned by researchers as influencing food intake and hence, nutritional status (Bartlett, 1998; Mobarhan & Trumbore, 1991; Thomas et al., 1991). Unfortunately, feeding ability was a primary focus in only four Level III studies (Berkhout et al., 1998; Du et al., 1993; Volicer et al., 1989; Wang et al., 1997) and one Level V study (Ott, Readman, & Backman, 1991) (see Table 3).

Berkhout et al. (1998) examined feeding disability (no, partial, total) in choosing food, bringing it to the mouth, chewing, and swallowing. After adjusting for age and gender, a significant relationship emerged, in the combined sample of nursing home residents with and without dementia, between body weight and the eating tasks. The group with no feeding disabilities had the highest body weight and the group with total disability had the lowest body weight. These relationships were more evident in existing than newly admitted residents and were strongest for bringing food to the mouth and chewing. Further, when feeding disability decreased over 2 years, body weight increased and when it increased, body weight decreased. No significant weight change was noted when feeding status remained constant.

Du et al. (1993) found a similar relationship in community dwelling subjects with mild to moderate AD. Correlations between changes in weight and feeding skills over a mean 2.9 years, as rated on the Blessed Dementia Rating Scale (BDRS) (Blessed, Tomlinson, & Roth, 1967) and the Record of Independent Living (Weintraub, 1986), suggested that as subjects required more assistance for feeding, their body weights decreased. No statistically significant relationship was found between change in body weight and duration or severity of dementia. The validity of the relationship between weight loss and self-feeding status was enhanced by the fact that other areas of self-care were not significantly related to weight loss.

Wang et al. (1997) found that on admission to long-term care, residents who were non-demented and independent in feeding had higher body weights than those who had dementia and required help with feeding. Due to the high intensity of nutrition-related services, most residents were able to maintain their weight during the 48-month study. Weight losses of more than 10 pounds were significantly more common among residents with dementia, especially those who were severely functionally impaired.

In their study of institutionalized subjects with AD, Volicer et al. (1989) used four classifications of feeding difficulties–fed self and fed by others which was subdivided into no feeding problems, refuses food, and chokes on food. Residents who fed themselves had less advanced dementia and had significantly higher body weight than those who were fed by others.

The Level V study by Ott et al. (1991) appraised the effectiveness of occupational therapy interventions for improving self-feeding in two subjects with dementia. An individualized occupational therapy program resulted in improvement in self-feeding skills and associated eating behaviors as well as increased dietary intake and body weight.

Although they did not include feeding status as a primary focus of their research, five of the previously examined studies used structured measures to grade feeding ability. Of the Level III (Franzoni et al., 1996; Singh et al., 1988) and Level V studies (Sandman et al., 1987), only Sandman et al. reported a difference in dietary intake of hospitalized patients between those who were and were not able to feed themselves (statistical significance was not reported). Rated on an unspecified

7-point feeding scale, subjects who were fed by others reportedly were not undernourished and consumed more calories than those who fed themselves. Results reported by Franzoni et al. with nursing home residents and Singh et al. with hospitalized patients, indicated that despite differences in feeding capabilities (as measured by the Barthel Index [Mahoney & Barthel, 1965]) and a 4-point scale (unaided: no problems, messily; aided: no problems, with difficulty), respectively, intake by subjects with dementia and those without was comparable.

The other two studies that used a structured feeding measure (Reyes-Ortega et al., 1997; White et al., 1996) reported no correlation between feeding skills and weight loss or other measures of nutrition. Reyes-Ortega et al. (Level V) did not provide adequate detail about their feeding assessment. White et al. (Level III) used BDRS data to rate functional and feeding (positive, negative) status. Although subjects lost more weight as their functional status deteriorated, no correlation was found between weight loss and feeding status.

Feeding ability is mentioned as an ancillary finding in other previously discussed studies. Most subjects in the studies by Suski and Nielsen (1989), Stähelin et al. (1983), and Winograd et al. (1991) were dependent in feeding. Suski and Nielson reported inadequate intake in subjects with severe dementia who were fed by others. In contrast, Stähelin et al. and Winograd et al. reported that their feeding dependent subjects with dementia had adequate dietary intakes. Stähelin et al. further reported that subjects maintained stable body weights and Winograd et al. reported that body weight and BMI of the subjects with dementia were not significantly different from the controls.

In summary, evidence from the five studies that identified self-feeding as a primary variable supports a relationship between self-feeding abilities and body weight. Those subjects who needed assistance to eat experienced greater variability in their body weights as well as a propensity to lose weight, while subjects who were able to feed themselves independently weighed more. In addition, a directional relationship was identified in three (Berkhout et al., 1998; Du et al., 1993; Ott et al., 1991) of the five studies such that as the subject's feeding abilities improved, their body weight increased and when feeding abilities deteriorated, body weight decreased. Adequate nutrition is fostered by the availability of appropriate caregiver support to assist with feeding disabilities (Ott et al., 1991; Wang et al., 1997). Finally, weight loss was not related to the duration or degree of dementia thereby supporting the notion that weight loss and undernutrition are not inevitable consequences of dementia.

Although stronger evidence is provided by studies where feeding status is a primary research variable, the findings from other studies should not be ignored. With the addition of these latter studies, the evidence linking impaired self-feeding skills and low dietary intake and/or low body weight becomes less definitive. Irrespective of feeding ability, no differences in dietary intake were discerned in either hospital (Singh et al., 1988) or nursing home (Franzoni et al., 1996) settings. Although no statistically significant relationship between overall self-care ability and weight loss was found in one study (Reyes-Ortega et al., 1997), overall functional status, but not feeding ability, was related to weight loss and change in another (White et al., 1996). In addition, dependence in feeding was related to both adequate (Sandman, 1987; Stähelin, 1983; Winograd, 1991) and inadequate (Suski & Nielson, 1989) nutritional intake.

DISCUSSION

Nutritional status can be measured by a variety of indicators–biochemical, anthropometric, dietary intake. Our review suggests that the detection of a significant relationship between dementia and undernutrition depends on the specific indicator. When nutritional status was measured by serum albumin levels (or other biochemical indices), there were generally no significant differences between subjects with and without dementia and values typically fell within normal ranges. When anthropometric measures of mid-arm and arm muscle circumference or triceps skinfold thickness were used as nutritional parameters, the detection of significant differences varied depending on the specific anthropometric measure, the site of subject residence (community-based, institutionalized), and the dementia diagnosis (AD versus MID and demented versus non-demented). When nutritional status was measured by weight change or body mass index, contradictory evidence emerged. Subjects with dementia tended to weigh less and have lower body mass indices than cognitively intact subjects, with these problems being particularly apparent for institutionalized subjects. Nonetheless, despite lower body weight, most studies reported that dietary intake in subjects with and without dementia was neither significantly different nor inadequate. In addition, nutritional indicators were related to independence and dependence in feeding as well as improvement and decline in self-feeding.

TABLE 3. Studies Addressing Self-Feeding Status in Relation to Nutritional Status

Study	Subject characteristics	Self-feeding measure	Nutrition measure	Results
Berkhout et al. (1998) Longitudinal design (2 years) Level III	With dementia • **Institutionalized** 145 women 55 AD; 20 MID; 70 other 46 men 17 AD: 13 MID: 16 other • Degree of dementia not reported Without dementia • **Institutionalized** 248 women 75 men Total Sample • Age—women (not differentiated by dementia): 83.0 years (existing Ss)* 81.6 years (new Ss)* • Age—men (not differentiated by dementia): 80.3 years (existing Ss)* 79.0 years (new Ss)*	3 level scale: No, Partial, Total disability. Rating considered choosing food, taking food to mouth, & chewing/swallowing.	Body weight	Ss with no feeding disability had highest body weight; Ss who were totally disabled for feeding had lowest body weight. Inability to take food to mouth & chew had highest correlation with weight loss. Male & female Ss with dementia who were residents at facility at study initiation weighed less than their newly admitted counterparts.
Du et al. (1993) Longitudinal design (5 year period/ mean 2.9 years) Level III	With dementia • **Community based** 50 women/ 31 men Sample age 69.0 ± 8.6 years. Blessed Dementia Rating Scale (BDRS) 21.0 ± 10.2 • None Without dementia	1 structured question (addressing cleanliness, appropriate utensil use, performance with finger foods, cutting & pouring), on BDRS and Record of Independent Living scored as "0, 1, 2, 3" with higher number reflecting greater impairment.	Body weight	High correlation between self-feeding ability & weight loss—as more assistance for feeding was needed (eating scores increased), weight decreased.

Study	Subject characteristics	Self-feeding measure	Nutrition measure	Results

Volicer et al. (1989)
 	
Cross-sectional design with longitudinal analysis of mortality (2 years)
 	
Level III
	<u>With dementia</u>
	• **Institutionalized**
	• 2 women/71 men
	• Independent feeders
	  69.7 ± 1.2 years
	  MMSE 4.6 ± 1.6
	• Dependent feeders
	  66.8 ± 1.0 years
	  MMSE 0.5 ± 0.4
	• Dependent feeders/Food refusal
	  70.5 ± 1.2 years
	  MMSE 0.3 ± 0.3
	• Dependent feeders/Choking
	  68.1 ± 1.4 years
	  MMSE 0.4 ± 0.2
	  <u>Without dementia</u>
	• None
		24 question survey completed by nurses identifying ability to self-feed, choking episodes, & behaviors associated with refusing food, wandering, chewing & swallowing ability.	Body weight
			Dietary intake
				Ss who self-fed had significantly higher body weights than those who were fed by others. Ss (with choking & food refusal behaviors) fed by others had higher (but not significant) dietary intake.

TABLE 3 (continued)

Study	Subject characteristics	Self-feeding measure	Nutrition measure	Results
Wang et al. (1997) Longitudinal design (4 year period/ mean 30 ± 15 months) for Ss with dementia; 44 ± 8 months for Ss without dementia Level III	<u>With dementia</u> • **Institutionalized** • 68 women / 11 men • 85.0 ± 5.4 years (severely impaired) 86.7 ± 5.5 years (less impaired) • MMSE 1.2 ± 3.3 (27 women & 4 men) 7.7 ± 10.0 (41 women & 7 men) <u>Without dementia</u> • **Institutionalized** • 18 women / 8 men • 86.7 ± 7.1 years • MMSE 28.5 ± 1.9	Katz Activities of Daily Living Scale used to score degree of independence. Feeding status rated as independent, needing help for meal set-up (cutting meat, buttering bread), or receives assistance in feeding. Feeding score considered as 1 of 6 self-care activities.	Body weight	All Ss maintained body weight. Ss without dementia who self-fed had higher mean weights on admission; weight loss equal to or greater than 10 pounds was more common in Ss with dementia, who needed some or total assistance for feeding.
Ott et al. (1991) Multiple baseline single subject design (about 52 days) Level V	<u>With dementia</u> • **Institutionalized** • 2 women / 97 & 85 years <u>Without dementia</u> • None	4 level scale describing "independence," "verbally guided," "physically assisted," & "dependent."	Body weight Dietary intake	Body weight & dietary intake increased as feeding independence increased.

Note: Age expressed as mean ± standard deviation, if reported; AD = Alzheimer's disease; MID = Multi-infarct dementia; MMSE = Mini-Mental State Examination, expressed as mean ± standard deviation, if reported; Ss = Subjects; * Ss characterized by "existing"—facility residents at time study initiated & "new"—admitted to facility after study initiated

In view of this research summary, one might be tempted to conclude that there is no relationship between dementia, nutritional status, and feeding status. However, this conclusion must be tempered by salient limitations of the available research. First, we lack comprehensive data about the emergence of undernutrition. Of the 19 studies reviewed, nine were cross-sectional in design or analyzed only weight or mortality longitudinally. As such, nutritional status was examined at only one point. To appreciate the emergence of undernutrition, that is to say, when it begins and how it progresses, longitudinal studies are essential. However, of the nine studies that examined nutritional indices longitudinally, time series data were available in only five (Barrett-Conner et al., 1996; Spindler et al., 1996; Wang et al., 1997; White et al., 1996; White et al., 1998), and with the exception of Spindler et al. (1996), were largely confined to body weight. Thus, the trajectory of nutritional status over the course of the studies, which extended from 6 months to 20 years, was not well documented. Comprehensive time series analyses tracing stability and change in cognitive status, biochemical parameters, anthropometric measures, dietary intake, and feeding status are lacking.

Second, we lack data about the interrelationships between dementia, nutrition, and feeding. No longitudinal study simultaneously examined the severity of dementia, adequacy of nutritional status, and level of feeding ability. The advent as well as the rate of decline may be different for each of these factors. We might postulate, for example, that increased cognitive impairment leads to difficulty feeding oneself, which in turn leads to loss of appetite, which in turn results in undernutrition, as evidenced in weight loss and lower body mass index. Thus, an intervention to alleviate feeding difficulties might slow the development of undernutrition. The intervention study conducted by Ott et al. (1991), where improvements were seen in self-feeding, dietary intake, and body weight following occupational therapy intervention, addressed this possibility.

Third, our review indicates that the research literature is virtually devoid of a randomized controlled trial of feeding interventions for people with dementia. The best available evidence comes from Level III studies, which support the tendency for people with dementia, living in the community or institutionalized, to weigh less and have lower body mass indices. The research evidence is less conclusive when dealing with other clinical measures of nutrition. Although the reasons and mechanisms responsible for weight loss are inconclusive, there is evidence to suggest that weight loss in people with dementia may be associated with decreases in the ability to self-feed. Thus, the hypothesis that weight loss and subsequent undernourishment are related to the pathophysiology of the dementia as suggested by Barrett-Connor et al. (1996), Reyes-Ortega et al. (1997), White et al. (1996), and White et al. (1998) remains to be tested.

Fourth, in the available evidence, the dementia-feeding-nutrition interrelationships were obscured by reliance on categorical measures of dementia (e.g., subjects with dementia versus without dementia). Further, even when dementia severity was systematically measured, through tools such as the Mini-Mental State Examination or the Clinical Dementia Rating Scale, dementia severity was used to describe the sample but was not analyzed in relation to problems in feeding or nutrition. Similar problems became apparent in regard to the feeding measures. Feeding was more often an ancillary than a primary focus of the studies, with a reliance on global (independent vs. dependent feeders; self fed vs. fed by others; able to feed vs. needs help) feeding measures.

The major purpose of this systematic review was to support the need for occupational therapy practitioners to take into account the influence that feeding interventions have on nutritional status, not just feeding independence. To accomplish this purpose, we recommend that measures of body weight and food intake be incorporated into the occupational therapy feeding assessment. Our recommendation of body weight is an obvious choice because of the association of weight loss with dementia progression. Our recommendation of food intake stems from the combination of several rationales: (1) changes in dietary intake are likely to precede changes in body weight; (2) changes in dietary intake secondary to feeding interventions may be positive (eat more foods) as well as negative (eat less food) and practitioners need to be sensitized to both potential outcomes; and, (3) dietary intake is a non-intrusive measure that can be readily observed during feeding intervention. Because weight and food intake measures are routinely taken in many health care settings, occupational therapy practitioners may elect to work collaboratively with nursing or dietary staff to obtain them.

As dementia progresses, the multiple cognitive and motor impairments that accompany decline contribute to performance deficits that frequently result in feeding disability. Our research review indicated that detection of a relationship between feeding and nutrition was in part dependent on the use of structured feeding instruments (Berkhout et al., 1998; Du et al., 1993; Ott et al., 1991; Volicer et al., 1989; Wang,

1997). Although the feeding measures used in these studies could be adopted by occupational therapy practitioners, our recommendation favors performance-based instruments often used in practice, such as the feeding item of the Klein-Bell scale (Klein & Bell, 1982). Alternatively, practitioners may wish to use the Refined ADL Assessment Scale (Tappen, 1997), which was devised specifically for clients with dementia. These measures are preferred over those used in previous research because they measure the components of feeding, not just overall feeding ability. Hence, they provide very specific data about feeding abilities that need to be reinforced, feeding disabilities that need to be targeted in intervention, and improvement secondary to intervention. The research also suggests that, in addition to transporting food to the mouth and chewing and swallowing, the task analysis for feeding assessment should include: choosing food, refusing food, choking, and using feeding utensils appropriately.

CONCLUSIONS AND RECOMMENDATIONS FOR QUALITY IMPROVEMENT STUDIES

Although undernutrition is common in people with dementia, it may not be an unavoidable consequence of disease progression. The evidence indicating that feeding performance in people with dementia can be improved, combined with the evidence that self-feeding status correlates with improved dietary intake and higher body weight, is critical information for occupational therapy practitioners, who are often responsible for addressing feeding issues in this population. The best evidence available suggests that occupational therapy feeding interventions can have an impact beyond that of task performance and are related to overall nourishment of people with dementia.

In the light of this evidence, there are multiple critical questions to be addressed by occupational therapy practitioners treating people with dementia who have performance deficits in self-feeding. These include: (1) Are self-feeding strategies currently used with people with dementia effective for enhancing self-feeding as well as maximizing food intake? (2) Of the strategies currently being used, which are most effective for promoting adequate food intake? (3) Does performance-based assessment identify subtle changes in feeding status that occur early in the dementing process that are commonly overlooked by self-report and informant-report methods? (4) Does a proactive or preventive approach (e.g., providing assistive devices for typical feeding deficits before feeding deficits actually occur) delay the development of feeding deficits? Studies that address these questions and include performance-based assessment of feeding and measures of nutritional status will enable occupational therapy practitioners to generate evidence-based practice guidelines and intervention protocols for enhancing self-feeding capabilities and promoting nutritional well-being in people with dementia. Equally as important, they will provide the outcome data necessary for justifying service provision and reimbursement.

REFERENCES

Amella, E.J., & the NICHE faculty (1998). Assessment and management of eating and feeding difficulties for older people: A NICHE protocol. *Geriatric Nursing, 19,* 269-275.

American Occupational Therapy Association (2000). Specialized knowledge and skills in eating and feeding for occupational therapy practice. *American Journal of Occupational Therapy, 54,* 629-640.

Barrett-Connor, E., Edelstein, S.L., Corey-Bloom, J., & Wiederholt, W.C. (1996). Weight loss precedes dementia in community-dwelling older adults. *Journal of the American Geriatrics Society, 44,* 1147-1152.

Bartlett, B.J. (1998). Factors associated with weight change in undernourished nursing home patients. *Journal of Rehabilitation Outcomes Measurement, 2* (6), 32-36.

Berkhout, A.M.M., Cools, H.J.M., & van Houwelingen, H.C. (1998). The relationship between difficulties in feeding oneself and loss of weight in nursing-home patients with dementia. *Age and Ageing, 27,* 637-641.

Berlinger, W.G., & Potter, J.F. (1991). Low body mass index in demented outpatients. *Journal of the American Geriatrics Society, 39,* 973-978.

Blessed, G., Tomlinson, B.E., & Roth, M. (1967). The association between quantitative measures of dementia and of senile changes in cerebral grey matter of elderly subjects. *British Journal of Psychiatry, 114,* 797-811.

Brunt, A.R., Schafer, E., & Oakland, M.J. (1999). Anthropometric measures of rural, elderly, community-dwelling women and the ability of the DETERMINE checklist to predict these measures. *Journal of Nutrition for the Elderly, 18* (3), 1-19.

Bucht, G., & Sandman, P.O. (1990). Nutritional aspects of dementia, especially Alzheimer's disease. *Age and Ageing, 19,* S32-36.

Burns, A., Marsh, A., & Bender, D.A. (1989). Dietary intake and clinical, anthropometric and biochemical indices of malnutrition in elderly demented patients and non-demented subjects. *Psychological Medicine, 19,* 383-391.

Chapman, K.M., & Nelson, R.A. (1994). Loss of appetite: Managing unwanted weight loss in the older patient. *Geriatrics, 49,* 54-59.

Clarke, D.M., Wahlqvist, M.L., & Strauss, B.J.G. (1998). Undereating and undernutrition in old age: Integrating bio-psychosocial aspects. *Age and Ageing, 27,* 527-534.

Du, W., DiLuca, C., & Growdon, J.H. (1993). Weight loss in Alzheimer's disease. *Journal of Geriatric Psychiatry and Neurology, 6,* 34-38.

Franklin, C.A., & Karkeck, J. (1989). Weight loss and senile dementia in an institutionalized elderly population. *Journal of the American Dietetic Association, 89,* 790-792.

Franzoni, S., Frisoni, G.B., Boffelli, S., Rozzini, R., & Trabucchi, M. (1996). Good nutritional oral intake is associated with equal survival in demented and nondemented very old patients. *Journal of the American Geriatrics Society, 44,* 1366-1370.

Gants, R. (1997). Detection and correction of underweight problems in nursing home residents. *Journal of Gerontological Nursing, 23* (12), 26-31.

Gilmore, S.A., Robinson, G., Posthauer, M.E., & Raymond, J. (1995). Clinical indicators associated with unintentional weight loss and pressure ulcers in elderly residents of nursing facilities. *Journal of the American Dietetic Association, 95,* 984-992.

Holm, M.B., Rogers, J.C., & James, A.B. (1998). Treatment of occupational performance areas. In M.E. Neistadt & E.B. Crepeau (Eds.), *Willard & Spackman's occupational therapy,* 9th ed. (pp. 323-364). Philadelphia: Lippincott.

Kerstetter, J.E., Holthausen, B.A., & Fitz, P.A. (1992). Malnutrition in the institutionalized older adult. *Journal of the American Dietetic Association, 92,* 1109-1116.

Klein, R.M., & Bell, B. (1982). Self-care skills: Behavior measurements with the Klein-Bell ADL Scale. *Archives of Physical Medicine and Rehabilitation, 63,* 335-338.

Lawton, M.P., & Brody, E.M. (1969). Assessment of older people: Self-maintaining and instrumental activities of daily living. *Gerontologist, 9,* 179-186.

Lutz, C.A., & Przytulski, K.R. (1997). *Nutrition and diet therapy* (2nd ed.). Philadelphia: F.A. Davis Company.

Mahoney, F.I., & Barthel, D.W. (1965). Functional evaluation: The Barthel index. *Maryland State Medical Journal, 14,* 61-65.

McKhann, G., Drachman, D., Folstein, M., Katzman, R., Price, D., & Stadlan, E.M. (1984). Clinical diagnosis of Alzheimer's disease: Report of the NINCDS-ADRDA work group under the auspices of Department of Health and Human Services task force on Alzheimer's disease. *Neurology, 34,* 939-944.

Mobarhan, S., & Trumbore, L.S. (1991). Nutritional problems of the elderly. *Clinics in Geriatric Medicine, 7,* 191-214.

Moore, A., McQuay, H., & Gray, J.A.M. (Eds.). (1995). Evidence-based everything. *Bandolier, 1* (12), 1.

Moore, M.C. (1997). *Pocket guide to nutritional care* (3rd ed.). Philadelphia: Mosby.

Morley, J.E. (1996). Dementia is not necessarily a cause of undernutrition. *Journal of the American Geriatrics Society, 44,* 1403-1404.

Morley, J.E., Thomas, D.R., & Kamel, H. (1998). Nutritional deficiencies in long-term care: Part I: Detection and diagnosis. *The Annals of Long-Term Care, 6* (Suppl. E), 1-12.

National Institute on Aging (1999). *Progress report on Alzheimer's Disease, 1999.* Bethesda, MD: National Institutes of Health.

Nightingale, J.M.D., Walsh, N., Bullock, M.E., & Wicks, A.C. (1996). Three simple methods of detecting malnutrition on medical wards. *Journal of the Royal Society of Medicine, 89,* 144-148.

Ott, F., Readman, T., & Backman, C. (1991). Mealtimes of the institutionalized elderly: A quality of life issue. *Canadian Journal of Occupational Therapy, 58,* 7-16.

Pierson, C.A. (1999). Ethnomethodologic analysis of accounts of feeding demented residents in long-term care. *Image: Journal of Nursing Scholarship, 31* (2), 127-131.

Reyes-Ortega, G., Guyonnet, S., Ousset, P.J., Nourhashemi, F., Vellas, B., Albarede, J.L., De Glizezinski, I., Riviere, D., & Fitten, L.J. (1997). Weight loss in Alzheimer's disease and resting energy expenditure (REE), a preliminary report. *Journal of the American Geriatrics Society, 45,* 1414-1415.

Sandman, P.O., Adolfsson, R., Nygren, C., Hallmans, G., & Winblad, B. (1987). Nutritional status and dietary intake in institutionalized patients with Alzheimer's disease and multiinfarct dementia. *Journal of the American Geriatrics Society, 35,* 31-38.

Silver, A.J. (1993). The malnourished older patient: When and how to intervene. *Geriatrics, 48,* 70-74.

Silver, A.J., Morley, J.E., Strome, S., Jones, D., & Vickers, L. (1988). Nutritional status in an academic nursing home. *Journal of the American Geriatrics Society, 36,* 487-491.

Simmons, S.F., & Reuben, D. (2000). Nutritional intake monitoring for nursing home residents: A comparison of staff documentation, direct observation, and photography methods. *Journal of the American Geriatrics Society, 48,* 209-213.

Singh, S., Mulley, G.P., & Losowsky, M.S. (1988). Why are Alzheimer patients thin? *Age and Ageing, 17,* 21-28.

Spindler, A.A., Renvall, M.J., Nichols, J.F., & Ramsdell, J.W. (1996). Nutritional status of patients with Alzheimer's disease: A 1-year study. *Journal of the American Dietetic Association, 96,* 1013-1018.

Stähelin, H.B., Hofer, H.O., Vogel, M., Held, C., & Seiler, W.O. (1983). Energy and protein consumption in patients with senile dementia. *Gerontology, 29,* 145-148.

Suski, N.S., & Nielsen, C.C. (1989). Factors affecting food intake of women with Alzheimer's type dementia in long-term care. *Journal of the American Dietetic Association, 89,* 1770-1773.

Tappen, R.M. (1997). *Interventions for Alzheimer's disease.* Baltimore: Health Professions Press.

Thomas, D.R., Kamel, H., & Morley, J.E. (1998). Nutritional deficiencies in long-term care: Part III: OBRA regulations and administrative and legal issues. *The Annals of Long-Term Care, 6* (12) (Suppl. November 1998), 1-9.

Thomas, D.R., Verdery, R.B., Gardner, L., Kant, A., & Lindsay, J. (1991). A prospective study of outcome from protein-energy malnutrition in nursing home residents. *Journal of Parenteral and Enteral Nutrition, 15,* 400-404.

Trombly, C.A. (1995). Retraining basic and instrumental activities of daily living. *Occupational therapy for physical dysfunction,* 4th ed. (pp. 289-318). Baltimore: Williams & Wilkins.

Volicer, L., Seltzer, B., Rheaume, Y., Karner, J., Glennon, M., Riley, M.E., & Crino, P. (1989). Eating difficulties in patients with probable dementia of the Alzheimer type. *Journal of Geriatric Psychiatry and Neurology, 2,* 188-195.

Wang, S.Y., Fukagawa, N., Hossain, M., & Ooi, W.L. (1997). Longitudinal weight changes, length of survival, and energy requirements of long term care residents with dementia. *Journal of the American Geriatrics Society, 45,* 1189-1195.

Watson, R. (1997). Undernutrition, weight loss and feeding difficulty in elderly patients with dementia: A nursing perspective. *Reviews in Clinical Gerontology, 7,* 317-326.

Watson, R. (1993). Measuring feeding difficulty in patients with dementia: Perspectives and problems. *Journal of Advanced Nursing, 18,* 25-31.

Weintraub, S. (1986). The record of independent living: An informant-completed measure of activities of daily living and behavior in elderly patients with cognitive impairment. *American Journal of Alzheimer Care, 1,* 35-39.

White, H., Pieper, C., & Schmader, K. (1998). The association of weight change in Alzheimer's disease with severity of disease and mortality: A longitudinal analysis. *Journal of the American Geriatrics Society, 46,* 1223-1227.

White, H., Pieper, C., Schmader, K., & Fillenbaum, G. (1996). Weight change in Alzheimer's disease. *Journal of the American Geriatrics Society, 44,* 265-272.

Winograd, C.H., Jacobson, D.H., Butterfield, G.E., Cragen, E., Edler, L.A., Taylor, B.S., & Yesavage, J.A. (1991). Nutritional intake in patients with senile dementia of the Alzheimer type. *Alzheimer Disease and Associated Disorders, 5,* 173-180.

Promoting Awareness and Understanding of Occupational Therapy and Physical Therapy in Young School Aged Children: An Interdisciplinary Approach

Keli Mu, PhD
Charlotte Royeen, PhD, OTR/L, FAOTA
Karen A. Paschal, PT, MS
Andrea M. Zardetto-Smith, PhD

SUMMARY. Public awareness and understanding of the professions of occupational therapy and physical therapy are limited. In this study, we examined perceptions of young school-aged children about occupational therapy and physical therapy as part of a larger grant project

Keli Mu is an Instructor in Department of Occupational Therapy, School of Pharmacy and Allied Health Professions.

Charlotte Royeen is Associate Dean for Research and Professor of Occupational Therapy, School of Pharmacy and Allied Health Professions.

Karen A. Paschal is Assistant Professor, Department of Physical Therapy, School of Pharmacy and Allied Health Professions.

Andrea M. Zardetto-Smith is Assistant Professor, Department of Pharmacy Sciences, School of Pharmacy and Allied Health Professions.

All are at Creighton University, 2500 California Plaza, Omaha, NE 68116 (E-mail: kmu@creighton.edu)

[Haworth co-indexing entry note]: "Promoting Awareness and Understanding of Occupational Therapy and Physical Therapy in Young School Aged Children: An Interdisciplinary Approach." Mu, Keli et al. Co-published simultaneously in *Occupational Therapy in Health Care* (The Haworth Press, Inc.) Vol. 15, No. 3/4, 2001, pp. 89-99; and: *Interprofessional Collaboration in Occupational Therapy* (ed: Stanley Paul, and Cindee Q. Peterson) The Haworth Press, Inc., 2001, pp. 89-99. Single or multiple copies of this article are available for a fee from The Haworth Document Delivery Service [1-800-HAWORTH, 9:00 a.m. - 5:00 p.m. (EST). E-mail address: getinfo@haworthpressinc.com].

89

funded by the National Institute on Drug Abuse (R25 DA12168 and R25 DA13522). One hundred three elementary school children (55 boys and 48 girls), grades 3 to 7, from local schools attended a one-day neuroscience and allied health profession exposition held at a local Boys & Girls Club. Children's understanding of occupational therapy and physical therapy was assessed through a pre/post questionnaire prior to and immediately after attending the exposition. At five of the 18 exhibition booths, faculty members and students from occupational therapy and physical therapy introduced and explained what occupational and physical therapists do at their work through interactive demonstrations. The results of the current study revealed that prior to attending the exposition, children's understanding of occupational therapy and physical therapy was limited. On pre-test, children reported they have some understanding of occupational therapy (18.6%) and physical therapy (34.9%). Children's understanding of occupational therapy and physical therapy, however, dramatically increased after the exposition (75.6% vs. 18.6%, 98.9% vs. 34.9%, respectively). Furthermore, the scope and depth of children's understanding also improved considerably. This finding suggests that an interactive neuroscience exposition including occupational therapy and physical therapy is an effective way to promote children's awareness and understanding of the professions. Implications for practice and future research directions are discussed in the study. *[Article copies available for a fee from The Haworth Document Delivery Service: 1-800-HAWORTH. E-mail address: <getinfo@ haworthpressinc.com> Website: <http://www.HaworthPress.com> © 2001 by The Haworth Press, Inc. All rights reserved.]*

KEYWORDS. Public perception of occupational therapy and physical therapy, school age children, awareness and understanding

INTRODUCTION

Occupational therapy and physical therapy are two prominent professions within allied health. Occupational therapy and physical therapy play significant roles in delivering effective health care treatment and services. In spite of the significant roles they play, public awareness and understanding of occupational and physical therapy are still limited. The general public, health care providers, and other professionals do not have a good understanding of occupational therapy and physical therapy (Brintnell, Madill, & Wood, 1981; Kallus, Noble, Bezner, &

Keely, 1999; Lee & Sheppard, 1998; Luna-Massey & Smyle, 1982; McAvoy, 1992; Royeen & Marsh, 1988; Smith, 1986; Yaniv, 1995). Practical experience and anecdotal evidence have revealed that if an individual is knowledgeable about occupational therapy or physical therapy, it is typically due to the fact that the individual, a family member, or a relative has received occupational therapy or physical therapy services.

The lack of public awareness and understanding of occupational therapy and physical therapy has been long recognized in both professions. Previous literature in occupational therapy has found consumers, health care administrators and other professionals do not have a clear and fully developed understanding of the roles and responsibilities of occupational therapists, even if they had received occupational therapy treatment or they had closely worked with occupational therapists (e.g., Brintnell, Madill, & Wood, 1981; McAvoy, 1992; Smith, 1986). In investigating patients' awareness of occupational therapists, McAvoy (1992) found that of 75 patients who had been seen previously by occupational therapists, 24 did not recall such contact. Brintnell and colleagues (1981) surveyed hospital administrators and other health care professionals in Alberta, Canada in order to understand their knowledge about occupational therapy's roles and functions. The results of their study suggested that although administrators and other allied health professionals have some knowledge about occupational therapy, their understanding and appreciation of the roles occupational therapists play in evaluating patients, developing treatment plans, and monitoring results were poor. Smith also found that physicians and nursing staff of medical wards lacked "either interest or understanding of the role of the occupational therapist in patient care" (p. 52).

The lack of full understanding of the roles and responsibilities of physical therapists has also been reported in the physical therapy literature (Kallus et al., 1999; Lee & Sheppard, 1998; Luna-Massey & Smyle, 1982; Sheppard, 1994). In particular, Sheppard (1994) found that the general public appeared to have a reasonably high awareness of musculosskeletal conditions treated by physical therapists. There appeared to be, however, a very low public awareness of the roles that physical therapists play in offering treatment in women's and children's conditions. In a subsequent study, Lee and Sheppard (1998) found that final year medical students were unaware or less aware of the involvement of physical therapists in managing Parkinson's disease, incontinence, asthma, and burns, etc., in spite of their high general knowledge about physical therapy.

Due to this lack of public awareness, both occupational therapy and physical therapy associations have undertaken efforts to increase public awareness and understanding of the professions. Specific and discrete strategies recommended in the literature to increase public awareness include offering open houses and awareness weeks, disseminating informational materials, using the full title of the profession as opposed to "OT" or "PT," establishing enthusiastic public relations, offering interdisciplinary education to other professions, and undertaking national awareness campaigns (Lee & Sheppard, 1998; McAvoy, 1992; Smith, 1986; Sheppard, 1994). Specifically in occupational therapy, the American Occupational Therapy Association (AOTA) has implemented a national campaign designed to increase public awareness and positive views of occupational therapy. This campaign has included advertising nationally in magazines such as *Redbook,* disseminating information about occupational therapy at state and local levels, building national coalitions, and increasing occupational therapy's profile through community oriented events like health fairs, open houses, and educational outreach activities.

Adults have been the primary targets of this public awareness campaign. Yet, comprehensive strategic planning needs a concomitant emphasis on children and adolescents including a focus on occupational therapy and physical therapy as possible career choices. Understanding these professions and the distinctions between them may further motivate children and adolescents to pursue educational and career choices based upon their own experiences. It is, therefore, important to disseminate information about occupational therapy and physical therapy not just to adults but also to children and adolescents. Not much is known, however, about children's perceptions of occupational therapy and physical therapy.

The study reported here is one study associated with a larger interdisciplinary grant project aimed at increasing the understanding of neuroscience and drug-abuse research by elementary-age school children. Specifically, this study examined and compared elementary school-aged children's perceptions of occupational therapy and physical therapy prior to, and following, exposure to an interactive demonstration of allied health professions that included occupational therapy and physical therapy.

METHOD

Neuroscience Exposition

The neuroscience exposition is a modified "reverse science fair." The concept of the "reverse science fair" was originated and pioneered by Colbern and a class of graduate students at the University of Illinois (Foundation for Biomedical Research, 1992; Zardetto-Smith et al., 2000). The Brains Rule! Neuroscience Exposition project is funded through the Science Education Drug Abuse Partnership Award program through the National Institute on Drug Abuse (R25 DA12168 and R25 DA13522). It aims to advance awareness about basic and applied neuroscience, and to promote public awareness and understanding of neuroscience and allied health professions including occupational therapy and physical therapy (Zardetto-Smith et al., 2000). This project takes an interdisciplinary approach in which neuroscientists and allied health professionals, such as occupational therapy, physical therapy, and pharmacy faculty members and students, work collaboratively to design and present neuroscience and health profession career projects to young school-aged children. Prior to the project event, professional participants attended an approximately two-hour long orientation meeting. During the orientation meeting, participants brainstormed, shared and discussed their ideas about presenting projects. During the actual events, presenters took turns visiting each exhibiting booth and learned from each other. After each the event, a debriefing meeting was held in which participants shared their comments and observation as well as what they learned from each other. Afterwards, recommendations for future similar events are proposed and discussed during these meetings.

Specific to the study reported here, a one-day event was held in the gym of a local Boys & Girls Club, the community partner. Faculty members and students of Creighton University, and the University of Nebraska Medical Center from neuroscience, medicine and allied health professions (e.g., occupational therapy, physical therapy, pharmacy, medical technology, etc.) presented their neuroscience and allied health profession projects to young school-aged children. Elementary school children, grades 3-7 from local schools, attended the exposition. The participating children formed small groups (5-6 children per group) and each group was led by a classroom teacher. The small groups took turns visiting each exhibition booth and adults presented their neuroscience and health profession projects to the children. Students' involvement was solicited during these presentations. Using evaluation forms specifically designed for children at the exposition, students evaluated the neuroscience and health profession projects at the end of each presentation. At the end of the day, the students were also asked to rank the presentations they had visited. Students' ranking was tallied and tabulated by project staff. The first, second and third place winners were awarded at the concluding gathering of the exposition.

Participants and Procedures

Participants. Of one hundred three (103) elementary school students, grades 3-7, who attended the neuroscience exposition, 55 were boys and 48 were girls (3rd grade, 2 students; 4th grade, 35 students; 5th grade, 46 students; 6th grade, 18 students; and 7th grade, 2 students). These students were recruited though administrators of the Boys & Girls Club from local elementary schools.

Measurements. A pre/post questionnaire was developed by the project team to assess children's knowledge and understanding of neuroscience and neuroscience-related professions, specifically occupational therapy and physical therapy. The questionnaire was an adaptation of one previously used by Colbern (http//: www.beemnet.com). The questionnaire asked what children think neuroscientists, occupational therapists, and physical therapists do in their careers.

Procedures. Specific to occupational therapy, faculty members and students from the Occupational Therapy Program in the School of Pharmacy and Allied Health Professions at Creighton University presented their projects to the children at three booths. In the health career booth, faculty from occupational therapy addressed what occupational therapists do in health care. The displayed equipment and devices at the booth included wheelchairs, crutches, pulling sock aids, etc. At the other two booths, various regions of the cerebral cortex were illustrated in terms of daily activities, and visiting children molded a brain out of "brain dough" to learn the major anatomical regions of the brain.

Faculty members and students from physical therapy presented projects related to physical therapy at two of the 18 booths. At one booth, adults introduced and explained what physical therapy is and what a physical therapist does at work through demonstration. The use of a therapy ball, wheelchair and other mobility aids such as walker and crutches in physical therapy were demonstrated in the booths, and students were encouraged to try on these devices and equipment. At the other booth, adults explained what vestibular dysfunction was and how one would feel if he or she had such dysfunction through simulation activities. Additionally, adults explained and demonstrated how a physical therapist assesses vestibular dysfunction.

Data analysis. Children's responses to the questionnaire were first categorized and tabulated and the percentages of responses in each category were then calculated. The response categories were generated by the research team members of the study through the constant comparison method (Bogdan & Biklen, 1992). Children's responses were analyzed by two team members separately. The two team members then met to review and compare their findings. When differences were noted, the two members reevaluated the data, and discussed the analysis until differences were resolved.

RESULTS

Of 103 children attending the exposition, 86 children completed the pre/post questionnaire. Only 86 sets of pre/post questionnaires were obtained since one group arrived after the pre-test due to a snowstorm. Additionally, some children left prior to the post-test questionnaire administration in the afternoon for various individual reasons.

Children's Perception of Occupational Therapy

On the pre-test, of 86 participating children, 30 children (30 out of 86, 34.9%) responded to the question *what do you think an occupational therapist does at work* and the remaining 56 children (65.1%) did not answer the question. Moreover, among those 30 children who responded, nearly half of the children (14 out of 30) answered: "I do not know." Categorization of children's responses yielded four categories and they were *helping others, similar to other professionals, do not know,* and *others.* Eleven participating children identified that occupational therapists help others and two children indicated that occupational therapists are counselors or physical therapists. Responses from three children fell into *others* category. On post-test, 67 (77.9%, 67 out of 86) answered the question *what do you think an occupational therapist does at work* while only 30 children (34.9%) answered on the pre-test. Among the 67 respondents, two children responded *I do not know.* Therefore, the majority of the children (75.6%, 65 out of 86) indicated that they have some understanding of occupational therapists, but only 16 children responded on the pre-test. Further analysis of children's responses yielded seven categories including *helping others* (42 children), *similar to other professionals* (3 children), *training or teaching others* (5 children), *identifying the working settings of occupational therapists* (2 children), *do not remember* (3 children), *do not know* (2 children), and *others* (10 children).

Children's Perception of Physical Therapy

On the pre-test, 39 out of 86 children (45.3%) answered the question *what do you think a physical therapist does at work* and the rest of the children (43.0%, 37 out of 86) did not answer the question. Among those 39 who responded, nine children answered: "I do not know." Thus, only a small percent of children (34.9%, 30 out of 86) reported they had some knowledge about physical therapy. Four response categories were generated from the data and these categories included *helps people to solve problems* (15 children out of 86 children), *fix and work on the body* (11 children), *do not know* (9 children) and *others* (4 children). On post-test, nearly all children (85 out of 86, 98.9%) answered the question *What do you think a physical therapist does at work?* Of 85 respondents, no children responded *I do not know.* It appeared that on the post-test, almost all children (98.9%) reported having knowledge and understanding about physical therapists whereas only a small percent of children (34.9%, 30 out of 86) reported so on pre-test. Five response categories were generated from post-test and they are *helps people to solve problems* (47 children), *fix and work on the body* (8 children), *teach others about the body* (10 children), *do not know* (11 children) and *others* (8 children).

DISCUSSION

This study examined and compared young school-aged children's understanding of occupational therapy and physical therapy prior to, and immediately following, attending a one-day exposition that interactively demonstrated the daily practice of occupational therapy and physical therapists. The major finding of the study is that prior to attending to the exposition, the majority of young school-aged children did not have ideas of what occupational therapy and physical therapy were. Only a small percent of the children reported they knew something about occupational therapy and physical therapy, 18.6% and 34.9% respectively.

Children's understanding of the professions of occupational therapy and physical therapy dramatically increased after attending the neuroscience exposition. Specific to occupational therapy, a vast majority of children (77.9%) were able to articulate what occupational therapists do at their work in comparison with only 18.6% prior to the exposition. The scope and depth of children's responses also considerably improved. Some insightful key words and concepts such as *reacher, instrument or device, motor skills, movement, self-function,* and *everyday things* emerged in children's responses. Similar improvement was also found in children's responses to physical therapy. After attending the exposition, almost all participating children (98.9%) reported that they had knowledge and understanding of what physical therapists do at their work. Furthermore, visual examination of the accuracy and complexity of children's responses by the authors of the study revealed that children's responses significantly improved. Some of the children's responses were "help people use devices to help people that can't use their body parts," "help you learn to walk after an injury," "they help people adapt to these injuries." Taken together, these findings suggest that efforts on the part of occupational therapists and physical therapists greatly enhance children's understanding of both professions.

In comparison with their understanding of physical therapy, children's knowledge about occupational therapy appears to be lower, even though there were more occupational therapy booths than physical therapy (3 booths from occupational therapy vs. 2 booths from physical therapy). This finding is in evidence both prior, and after, children attended the exposition. It appears physical therapy has a higher public image and awareness than occupational therapy. This finding is consistent with the author's general experience in education and practice.

Consistent with previous literature, this study also found that there is some confusion about the perception of the profession of occupational therapy. Occupational therapy may be perceived as the profession that helps others find jobs. Occupational therapists are often confused with other professionals such as physical therapists, social workers or school counselors. Such confusion and misunderstanding persisted in some of the children even after they attended the exposition. Effective strategies and further efforts are needed to explore and undertake to promote accurate understanding of occupational therapy.

Several limitations exist in this study which may limit the generality of the findings. The sample of the study was convenient and restricted to one geographical region. Further investigation needs to involve a larger sample from different geographical regions. Second, this study only focused on the quantity of children's responses, and the quality of children's responses (e.g., accuracy and complexity) was not formally analyzed. Further studies are needed to investigate children's responses both quantitatively and qualitatively. Finally, the number and the structure of exhibition booths from occupational therapy and physical therapy were not the same in the study. How such a discrepancy impacts the results of the study warrants further investigation.

CONCLUSION

In conclusion, this study illustrates how an interactive and interdisciplinary approach can increase awareness and understanding of school-aged children about allied health professions. In addition to increasing children's awareness of these professions, the exposition approach provides an opportunity for neuroscience professionals involved in basic research and clinical aspects of neuroscience (especially rehabilitative processes) to interact with one another. The exposition accomplishes this very effectively in a number of ways. The presenters are both faculty and students, so the students have an opportunity to act with established professionals in a community setting, much as they will later on in clinical clerkships or rotations. In clinical or research settings (even basic research) there is a renewed emphasis on interdisciplinary collaborations in either treatment or experimental approaches. This is particularly valuable, then, for the students who may have to participate in such collaborative paradigms some time in their careers. Secondly, during a follow-up meeting, the presenters themselves report that they have learned and gained more understanding of other health care professions at each event. This is facilitated by the presenters having the opportunity to view each other's activities, and the opportunity to intermingle on an informal basis during snack and lunch breaks. Indeed, the schedule of the event is set to provide opportunities for such interactions among the presenters to occur. Lastly, the positive experiences of the presenters have reinforced the value of this type of educational outreach as service to their respective professions as well as the community, thus providing good incentives to participate in similar future efforts.

AUTHOR'S NOTE

This study was supported by NIDA SEDAPA R25 DA12168 and R25 DA13522 awarded to Creighton University. The authors are grateful to the children and administration of the Boys & Girls Club of Omaha. Our thanks also go to the faculty and students from Creighton University and the University of Nebraska Medical Center for their enthusiastic participation.

REFERENCES

Bogdan, R., & Biklen, S. K. (1992). *Qualitative research for education: An introduction to theory and methods* (2nd. Ed.). Needlam Heights: Allyn and Bacon.

Brintnell, E. S., Madill, H. M., & Wood, P. A. (1981). What do they think we do? O.T. functions as perceived by administrators and allied health professionals. *Canadian Journal of Occupational Therapy, 48* (2), 76-82.

Foundation for Biomedical Research (1992). Interview: Helping kids get a feel for science. *The Foundation for Biomedical Research Newsletter, 9,* 4-6.

Kallus, K., Noble, D., Bezner, J., & Keely, G. (1999). An assessment of high school student's knowledge of physical therapy and the factors that influence their knowledge. *Journal of Physical Therapy Education, 13,* 4-11.

Lee, K., & Sheppard, L. (1998). An investigation into medical students' knowledge and perception of physiotherapy services. *Australian Physiotherapy, 44,* 239-245.

Luna-Massey, P., & Smyle, L. (1982). Attitudes of consumers of physical therapy in California toward the professional image of physical therapists. *Physical Therapy, 62,* 309-314.

McAvoy, E. (1992). Occupational Who? Never heard of them! An audit of patient awareness of occupational therapists. *British Journal of Occupational Therapy, 55,* 229-232.

Royeen, C. B., & Marsh, D. (1988). Promoting occupational therapy in the schools. *The American Journal of Occupational Therapy, 42,* 713-717.

Sheppard, L. (1994). Public perception of physiotherapy: Implications for marketing. *Australian Physiotherapy, 40,* 265-271.

Smith, L. A. (1986). How do other professions view occupational therapy? *British Journal of Occupational Therapy, 49* (2), 51-52.

Yaniv, L. (1995). Our public image. *OT Week, 9* (37), 22-23.

Zardetto-Smith, A., Mu, K., Ahmad, O., & Royeen, C. B. (2000). A model program for bringing neuroscience to children: An informal neuroscience education program bridges a gap. *The Neuroscientist, 6,* 159-168.

Collaboration Between Team Members
in Inclusive Educational Settings

Susan M. Nochajski, PhD, OTR/L

SUMMARY. The inclusion of students with disabilities into general education settings and programs has necessitated the development of integrated, collaborative service delivery models that are compatible with the goals and purpose of inclusive education. Although there is considerable theoretical literature on collaboration, there is minimal empirical data available on the process or its outcomes. The purpose of this exploratory study was to gain insight on the perspectives of regular and special educators, and occupational, physical, and speech-language therapists towards collaboration. Using a semi-structured interview, participants (n = 51) responded to questions concerning the definition, nature, and extent of collaboration in their school setting. Participants also responded to questions related to the advantages of, barriers towards, and strategies to promote collaboration. Participants typically defined collaboration as not a problem-solving process, but in terms of activities associated with it. Results indicate that participants believed collaboration was mutually beneficial for both students and team members. However, implementing a collaborative approach was problematic. Lack of administrative approval for time for planning meetings was the most frequently cited barrier to collaboration. Although 51.6% of the participants reported time available

Susan M. Nochajski is affiliated with the University at Buffalo, Department of Occupational Therapy, 515 Kimball Tower, Buffalo, NY 14214.

[Haworth co-indexing entry note]: "Collaboration Between Team Members in Inclusive Educational Settings." Nochajski, Susan M. Co-published simultaneously in *Occupational Therapy in Health Care* (The Haworth Press, Inc.) Vol. 15, No. 3/4, 2001, pp. 101-112; and: *Interprofessional Collaboration in Occupational Therapy* (ed: Stanley Paul, and Cindee Q. Peterson) The Haworth Press, Inc., 2001, pp. 101-112. Single or multiple copies of this article are available for a fee from The Haworth Document Delivery Service [1-800-HAWORTH, 9:00 a.m. - 5:00 p.m. (EST). E-mail address: getinfo@haworthpressinc.com].

101

for collaborative planning by regular and special educators, only 21.5% of the participants reported this time being available for therapists to meet with educators. Education about collaboration, either in professional/preservice education programs or as continuing education, was recommended as a strategy to facilitate a collaborative approach. Although a collaborative approach is being used by therapists and educators more and more frequently, there is a need for research to validate its efficacy. *[Article copies available for a fee from The Haworth Document Delivery Service: 1-800-HAWORTH. E-mail address: <getinfo@haworthpressinc.com> Website: <http://www.HaworthPress.com> © 2001 by The Haworth Press, Inc. All rights reserved.]*

KEYWORDS. Collaboration, special education, occupational therapy, related services

Inclusion has frequently been referred to as being among the "best practices" in the education of students with disabilities (Gartner & Lipsky, 1987; Reynolds, Wang, & Wolberg, 1987; Will, 1986). Although not all persons in the educational community advocate for this practice (Jenkins, Pious, & Jewell, 1990), students with disabilities are being included in regular education in increasing numbers. As a result, the inclusion of students with disabilities into general education settings and programs has necessitated the development and restructuring of service delivery models that are compatible with the goals and purposes of inclusive education (Swenson, 2000). The model of service delivery traditionally used in educational settings, specifically, multidisciplinary teams where students with disabilities receive special education and related services outside the regular education classroom, does not foster inclusive education. Educational teams have recognized that a more integrated approach to service delivery must be adopted (Rainforth, York, & Macdonald, 1992).

In a more inclusive and integrated approach to the education of students with disabilities, the regular educator has overall responsibility for the education of all students, including those with disabilities (Alper & Ryndak, 1992). However, responsibility for the design and implementation of the curriculum is shared between the regular and special educator (Falvey, Coots, Bishop, & Grenot-Scheyer, 1989). Similarly, therapies must be integrated into the educational program and therapists into the classroom (York, Rainforth, & Giangreco, 1990). Collaboration is an essential component of providing integrated educational programs for students with disabilities.

Rainforth, York, and Macdonald (1992) define collaboration as a "process of problem solving by team members, each of whom contributes his or her knowledge and skills and is viewed as having equal status" on the team (p. 11). It is also viewed as a process involving all team members in order to achieve shared goals for students and requires a willingness to share knowledge, expertise, and responsibility for organizing, planning and implementing educational programs (Swenson, 2000).

Collaboration between regular and special education teachers is a practice widely acknowledged as being important and facilitating the success of students with disabilities (Reeve & Hallahan, 1994; Voltz, Elliott, & Cobb, 1994). Likewise, collaboration between educators and related service providers such as occupational and physical therapists, and speech-language pathologists is equally as important. However, the recognition of the benefits of collaboration does not necessarily result in collaborative practices (Rainforth, York, & Macdonald, 1993). Voltz, Elliott, and Cobb (1994) found significant differences between the ideal perception of collaboration and the actual collaboration experienced by regular and special educators. There is little, if any, research that addresses therapists' perceptions of collaboration.

The purpose of this study, which is descriptive and exploratory in nature, is to gain insight on the perspectives towards collaboration of regular and special educators, and occupational, physical, and speech-language therapists working with students with disabilities in inclusive educational settings.

METHOD

Participants

Convenience sampling was used to select school districts and five school districts in western New York were involved in this study. Each of the school districts selected included students with disabilities into regular education programs. Student disabilities included: (a) learning disabilities; (b) cerebral palsy; (c) multiple physical disabilities with cognitive impairment; (d) developmental delay; (e) Down Syndrome; and (f) emotional/behavioral disorders. Two of the school districts were rural, two were suburban, and one was urban.

Participants (n = 51) included regular educators (n = 17), special educators (n = 12), occupational therapists (n = 7), physical therapists (n = 7) and speech-language pathologists (n = 8). Table 1 depicts information about the number of years of work experience of the participants.

Data Collection and Analysis

A semi-structured interview was used in this study. Interviews with participants typically lasted between 20 and 30 minutes and were audiotaped for later transcription. Guiding questions for the interview included:

1. What is meant by collaboration in your school setting;
2. To what extent is there collaboration between educators and therapists and between regular and special educators in your school setting;
3. What do you see as the advantages of collaboration;
4. What do you see as the barriers towards collaboration;
5. How could collaboration be improved in your school setting?

The transcribed interviews were analyzed and coded to determine general descriptive categories for responses. These responses are reported as the percentage of participants giving that description.

TABLE 1. Mean, Range and Standard Deviation for Years of Work Experience

	Mean (in years)	Range (in years)	Standard Deviation (in years)
Regular Educators (n = 17)	10.65	1-30	8.90
Special Educators (n = 12)	12.67	3-25	6.79
Occupational Therapists (n = 7)	5.71	1-10	3.73
Physical Therapists (n = 7)	8.29	4-18	5.19
Speech-Language Pathologists (n = 8)	6.62	3-11	2.56

RESULTS

Definition of Collaboration

Participants, often those working within the same school, provided varied descriptions of collaboration to explain their understanding of the concept as used in their school setting. Communication and coordination, important aspects of collaboration, were terms used to describe collaboration by 92.1% and 74.5% of the participants, respectively. However, none of the participants offered a formal definition of collaboration; rather, as can be seen in Table 2, they explained the concept in terms of activities they perceived to be associated with collaboration, such as using a transdisciplinary approach and integrating services.

Participants who were either therapists or special educators provided descriptions using these terms; none of the regular educators used this terminology in their descriptions of collaboration. A relatively small percentage of participants (3.9%) referred to problem solving, a major purpose of collaboration, in their descriptions. Although consultation and collaboration refer to different approaches, 21.6% of the participants viewed them as being synonymous.

TABLE 2. Participants' Definition of Collaboration

Description	Percentage of Participants Reporting
Communicating better with team members	92.1%
Coordinating efforts	74.5%
All team members working on the same goals and objectives	66.6%
Using a transdisciplinary approach	64.7%
Integrating services/"push-in" rather than "pull out"	58.8%
Equal roles and responsibilities for regular and special educators; sharing responsibility for the students' education	29.4%
Sharing of expertise between all individuals working with the student	23.5%
Consulting with specialists	21.6%
Increased involvement of family in planning and decision making	15.7%
Problem solving process	3.9%

Extent and Type of Collaboration

All participants stated that they collaborated with other members of the educational team. However, as collaboration was defined differently by the participants, the nature of collaboration experienced by the participants varied considerably. Table 3 illustrates the nature and frequency of collaboration as perceived by the participants.

All participants appeared to regard any type of discussion about a student, either formal or informal, as being collaboration. Discussion and planning were two descriptions provided by the participants related to the type of collaboration occurring at their school setting. Approximately 60% of the participants attended monthly team meetings at which time students were discussed; 13.7% attended bimonthly team meetings and 9.8% weekly team meetings. However, the number of participants reporting attending meetings with other team members to specifically plan teaching strategies and class activities in general or for specific student needs was significantly lower. Approximately half of the regular and special educators met on either a monthly or weekly basis to plan; however, only 21.5% of the participants reported monthly planning sessions that involved educators and therapists, and none of the participants reported weekly planning meetings between educators and therapists.

TABLE 3. Type or Extent of Collaboration

Type or Extent of Collaboration	Percentage of Participants Reporting
Daily informal discussions (hall, lunchroom, parking lot)	100%
Monthly team meetings to **discuss** students	60.7%
Monthly **planning** meetings for regular and special educators	37.9%
Monthly **planning** meetings for educators and therapists	21.5%
Bimonthly team meetings to **discuss** students	13.7%
Weekly **planning** meetings for regular and special educators	13.7%
Weekly team meetings to **discuss** students	9.8%
Weekly **planning** meetings for educators and therapists	0%

Advantages or Benefits of Collaboration

Participants viewed collaboration as being beneficial for both students and team members. As can be seen in Table 4, a significant majority of participants (86.2%) viewed collaboration as being beneficial in facilitating students' progress and enabling them to meet their educational goals. Similarly, 80.3% of the participants stated that collaboration would be instrumental in enabling team members to learn from the knowledge, expertise, and experience of others on the team. Thirty-seven percent of the participants, the majority of whom were regular educators, suggested that collaboration would likely result in therapists being viewed as more vital, important team members.

Barriers Toward Implementing Collaboration

Although collaboration was perceived to have benefits and advantages for both students and team members, participants, none the less, noted numerous barriers towards implementing a collaborative approach. These barriers are listed in Table 5.

Participants (88.2%) most frequently cited lack of administrative support, indicated by administrators either not providing any or enough time for educators and therapists to meet, as a barrier towards a collaborative approach. The second most frequently cited barrier was the lack of a consistent presence of therapists at the school. Approximately 82% of the participants stated that the itinerant role of the related service pro-

TABLE 4. Advantages of Collaboration

Advantage or Benefit of Collaboration	Percentage of Participants Reporting
Student benefits/makes progress/achieves goals when the team works together	86.2%
Team members learn from the knowledge, expertise, and experience of others on the team	80.3%
Teachers and therapists working together	62.7%
Integrated education plan for the student	56.8%
Therapists more likely to be viewed as vital team members	37.2%
Regular and special educators have equivalent roles	19.6%

TABLE 5. Barriers Toward Implementing a Collaborative Approach

Barrier	Percentage of Participants Reporting
Lack of administrative support (no time/not enough time allowed for planning/meeting)	88.2%
Lack of consistent presence of therapists on site	82.3%
Too time consuming	76.4%
Lack of knowledge regarding the expertise of other professionals	43.1%
Lack of interaction by regular educators with the inclusion students	27.4%
Lack of clear role delineation	25.4%
Special educators provide too much support; are too "involved"	17.6%
Lack of administrative understanding of inclusion and the need for collaboration	17.6%
Philosophical differences towards education of students with disabilities	15.6%
Little communication between regular educators and other team members	13.7%
Loss of professional identity for special educators	9.8%
Personality conflicts between team members	7.8%

viders, not being at the school on a daily basis and only spending a portion of each day when there, made it extremely difficult for collaboration to take place. This also made it more difficult for educators to gain an understanding of how the various therapies helped the students to progress academically. A large percentage of participants (76.4%) felt that collaboration was just too time consuming and intensive and were not convinced that the benefits outweighed the costs.

Interestingly, 27.4% of the participants, the majority of whom were special educators, stated that a lack of interaction by regular educators with the inclusion students was a barrier to collaboration. Conversely, 17.6% of the participants, the majority of whom were regular educators, suggested that special educators were too involved and provided too much support to students with disabilities who were included in their regular education classrooms.

Strategies to Promote Collaboration

Participants offered several suggestions as to how collaboration could be improved. As can be seen in Table 6, there seemed to be a consensus among participants regarding the strategies to be used; each strategy was suggested by over 50% of the participants.

Participants thought more knowledge about collaboration would be extremely useful in promoting its use. Approximately 86% of the participants responded that attending continuing education or in-service training on collaboration would be helpful. However, 78.4% also reported that administrative support, including release time for continuing education, is also needed. Participants (78.4%) also thought that more information about collaboration, team process and team member roles and responsibilities was needed in professional or preservice educational programs.

In an effort to promote better and more effective collaboration, participants (80.3%) also suggested a need for improved communication between regular and special educators and advocated for therapy to be provided in the classroom (56.8%).

DISCUSSION

The results of this study suggest that there is a considerable difference in theory and practice in regard to collaboration in inclusive educational settings. While educators and therapists believe collaboration is

TABLE 6. Strategies Suggested by Participants to Improve Collaboration

Strategy	Percentage of Participants Reporting
Inservices and continuing education related to collaboration	86.2%
Improve communication between regular and special educators	80.3%
Include more on collaboration in professional/preservice educational programs	78.4%
Administrative support (i.e., time for planning; more release time for continuing education)	76.4%
Increased staffing (i.e., more therapists on site)	64.7%
Provide therapy services in the classroom	56.8%

mutually advantageous for both students and team members, it does not appear that a true collaborative approach is being used by the teams of the participants in this study.

Participants did not seem to have a clear understanding of the concept of collaboration and defined much of what was occurring at their schools as collaboration when it appears to have been something else. Lawson and Sailor (2000) suggest "when a new cottage industry develops around a bewildering array of buzzwords, something important is happening" (p. 1). Clearly, collaboration is a key and essential component of inclusive educational programs but it was not well understood by the participants in this study. They used a variety of "buzzwords" to describe the concept: trans-disciplinary approach, integrated services, coordinating efforts, parental involvement, consultation. A significantly small percentage of the participants (3.9%) viewed collaboration as a problem-solving process as defined by Rainforth, York and Macdonald (1992), yet almost 22% of the participants equated collaboration with consulting with specialists. Consulting implies a hierarchy in that team members are seeking advice from an "expert" whereas collaboration views all team members as having equal status (Rainforth, York, & Macdonald, 1992).

According to Gardner (1994), a collaborative climate is one in which people work well together and have clear roles and responsibilities. In reporting the perceived barriers towards collaboration, participants in this study suggest that a collaborative climate is lacking in their educational settings. Almost half of the participants (43.1%) reported a lack of knowledge about the expertise of other professionals and 25.4% indicated a lack of clear role delineation. Overall, the regular educators were not familiar with the contributions that therapists could make to the educational process. Responses of the participants suggested that team members might not work together as well as would be necessary to facilitate collaboration. Personality conflicts between team members were reported as a barrier to collaboration by 7.8% of the participants. Additionally, participants were concerned with the philosophical differences of team members towards the education of students with disabilities (15.6%), felt there was little communication between regular educators and other team members (13.7%), and that collaboration might result in a loss of professional identity for special educators (9.8%).

Participants offered several strategies to facilitate a collaborative approach. Education, both in professional/preservice educational programs and as continuing education or in-service training, was suggested by over 80% of the participants. Collaboration is a relatively new term in the inclusion, special education, and related services literature (Swenson, 2000). Since many of the participants have over ten years of work experience, it is likely that collaboration was not a topic in their professional training programs, resulting in their lack of understanding of the concept.

On a positive note, over 80% of the participants viewed collaboration as a means for team members to learn from the knowledge, expertise, and experience of others. Lawson and Sailor (2000) characterize this as "enlightened self-interest" (p. 18) and suggest that as a result the professional has a vested interest in the collaborative undertaking. Collaboration continues when all parties involved benefit from it.

Over 80% of the participants also reported that student progress and attainment of educational goals was an advantage of collaboration. It has been suggested that educators and health-related service providers often get caught up "in just another in a long line of human service bandwagons" without an empirical base of support (Giangreco, York, & Rainforth, 1989, p. 5). This is also happening with collaboration. Although there is a substantial amount of literature about the process of collaboration, little is known about its effectiveness or its impact on outcomes for students with disabilities. While it is often a professional's intuitive belief that collaboration is an effective method of service delivery, there has been little research investigating collaboration among team members in inclusive educational settings. This study provides some preliminary descriptive data regarding the perceptions of educators and therapists towards collaboration in inclusive educational settings; further experimental research is needed.

REFERENCES

Alper, S., & Ryndak, D.L. (1992). Educating students with severe handicaps in regular classes. *Elementary School Journal, 92* (3), 373-387.

Falvey, M., Coots, J., Bishop, K., & Grenot-Scheyer, M. (1989). Educational and curriculum adaptations. In S. Stainback, W. Stainback, & M. Forest (Eds.). *Educating all students in the mainstream of regular education* (pp. 143-158). Baltimore: Paul H. Brookes Publishing Company.

Garner, H.G. (1994). Critical issues in teamwork. In H.G. Garner & F.P. Orelove (Eds.). *Teamwork in human services: Models and applications across the life span* (pp. 1-18). Newton, MA: Butterworth-Heinemann.

Gartner, A., & Lipsky, D. (1987). Beyond special education: Toward a quality system for all students. *Harvard Educational Review, 57,* 367-395.

Giangreco, M., York, J., & Rainforth, B. (1989). Providing related services to learners with severe handicaps in educational settings: Pursuing the least restrictive environment. *Pediatric Physical Therapy, 1* (2), 55-63.

Jenkins, J., Pious, C., & Jewell, M. (1990). Special education and the regular education initiative: Basic assumptions. *Exceptional Children, 56,* 479-491.

Lawson, H.A., & Sailor, W. (2000). Integrating services, collaborating, and developing connections with schools. *Focus on Exceptional Children, 33* (2), 1-XX.

Rainforth, B., York, J., & Macdonald, C. (1992). *Collaborative teams for students with severe disabilities.* Baltimore: Paul H. Brookes Publishing Company.

Reeve, P.T., & Hallahan, D.P. (1994). Practical questions about collaboration between general and special educators. *Focus on Exceptional Children, 26* (7), 1-10.

Reynolds, M., Wang, M., & Wolberg, H. (1987). The necessary restructuring of special and regular education. *Exceptional Children, 53,* 391-398.

Swenson, N.C. (2000). Comparing traditional and collaborative settings for language interventionists. *Communications Disorders Quarterly, 22* (1), 12-XX.

Voltz, D.L., Elliott, R.N., & Cobb, H.B. (1994). Collaborative teacher roles: Special and general educators. *Journal of Learning Disabilities, 27* (8), 525-527.

Will, M. (1986). Educating children with learning problems: A shared responsibility. *Exceptional Children, 53,* 411-416.

Wood, M. (1998). Whose job is it anyway? Educational roles in inclusion. *Exceptional Children, 64* (2), 181-195.

York, J., Rainforth, B., & Giangreco, M.F. (1990). Trans-disciplinary teamwork and integrated therapy: Clarifying the misconceptions. *Pediatric Physical Therapy,* (2), 73-79.

A Response to Traumatized Children: Developing a Best Practices Model

Yvette D. Hyter, PhD, CCC-SLP
Ben Atchison, PhD, OTR
James Henry, MSW, PhD,
Mark Sloane, DO
Connie Black-Pond, MA, CSW, LPC

SUMMARY. This manuscript describes the key components for establishing collaborative partnerships in the delivery of services to children who have been traumatized by abuse, neglect, and prenatal exposure to alcohol. Specifically, the manuscript addresses: the national need for such collaborative partnerships; the effects of abuse, neglect, and prenatal exposure to alcohol on developmental and educational outcomes; the process used to develop the children's trauma assessment center (CTAC) including discussion on the family centered and transdisciplinary nature of the center; and the accomplishment and future goals of CTAC. The members of the CTAC team currently include the disciplines of counseling, occupational therapy, pediatric medicine, social work, and speech-language pathology. Future goals include expanding the core team to include the nursing and educational psychology disciplines. *[Article copies available for a fee from The Haworth Document Delivery Service: 1-800-HAWORTH. E-mail address: <getinfo@haworthpressinc.com> Website: <http://www.HaworthPress.com> © 2001 by The Haworth Press, Inc. All rights reserved.]*

Yvette D. Hyter, Ben Atchison, James Henry, Mark Sloane, and Connie Black-Pond are affiliated with Western Michigan University, Southwestern Michigan Children's Trauma Assessment Center, 1000 Oakland Drive, 3rd floor, Kalamazoo, MI 49008.

[Haworth co-indexing entry note]: "A Response to Traumatized Children: Developing a Best Practices Model." Hyter, Yvette D. et al. Co-published simultaneously in *Occupational Therapy in Health Care* (The Haworth Press, Inc.) Vol. 15, No. 3/4, 2001, pp. 113-140; and: *Interprofessional Collaboration in Occupational Therapy* (ed: Stanley Paul, and Cindee Q. Peterson) The Haworth Press, Inc., 2001, pp. 113-140. Single or multiple copies of this article are available for a fee from The Haworth Document Delivery Service [1-800-HAWORTH, 9:00 a.m. - 5:00 p.m. (EST). E-mail address: getinfo@haworthpressinc.com].

KEYWORDS. Transdisciplinary assessment, family centered services, abuse, neglect, prenatal exposure to alcohol

Children who are traumatized by abuse, neglect, and/or prenatal exposure to alcohol are at high-risk for significant developmental delays across many domains including behavioral, communication, educational, emotional, physical, and psychological development (Avery, 1994; Chasnoff, 2000; Dale, Kendall, Humber, & Sheehan, 2000; Dore, 1999; Ford, Racusin, Ellis, Davis, Reiser, Fleischer, & Thomas, 2000; Nash, Hulsey, Sexton, Harralson, & Lambert, 1993; Perry, 1999a, 1999b; Streissguth, 1999; Terr, 1991; Turpin, 1993; Young, 1993). When multiple issues simultaneously occur, the symptoms are complex and require complex and multi-layered solutions. Moreover, these children do not develop in a vacuum; therefore, their development, or lack thereof, should be considered in the context of their environment (Foley, 1990). Consequently, the assessments and interventions offered to these children must consider the interaction between familial, social, and individual factors to determine the depth and range of potential risk, and to determine the best solutions to reduce or address that risk (Hummel & Prizant, 1993; Nelson, 1998).

The Southwestern Michigan Children's Trauma Assessment Center (CTAC) was developed in response to the need for comprehensive services for children who have been traumatized by abuse, neglect, and/or prenatal exposure to alcohol (i.e., referred to from now on as traumatized children). CTAC is designed to provide comprehensive, transdisciplinary team-based assessments of traumatized children, of whom 75% are in out-of-home placements (i.e., with relatives, adoptive families, or in foster care). The transdisciplinary team consists of faculty and other professions from the disciplines of Counseling, Occupational Therapy, Pediatrics, Social Work, and Speech-Language Pathology. The purpose of this article is to describe the evolution of this transdisciplinary team to meet the needs of traumatized children. Following a review of the pertinent literature, which indicates the national need for a center such as CTAC, the primary components to develop our program are described including the results of a needs survey, development of the transdisciplinary team of professionals, the assessment protocol, and future program goals.

THE NATIONAL NEED FOR CTAC

In the United States, an increasing number of children experience trauma resulting from abuse and/or neglect (National Committee to Prevent Child Abuse [NCPCA], 1995). Child abuse is any behavior directed at a child that jeopardizes or damages the child's physical, mental, or emotional health and development (National Council on Child Abuse & Family Violence [NCCAFV] 1999). Neglect is the continued failure to provide necessary and appropriate care and protection such as food, shelter, clothing, and medical care (Gaudin, 1993; NCCAFV, 1999). Reports of child abuse and neglect (i.e., child maltreatment) increased at the alarming rate of 63% between 1985 and 1994 (NCPCA, 1995). Approximately 5 million children experience some type of trauma each year (Perry, 1999, 2000) and 2.5 to 3 million of those children experience physical and/or sexual abuse and neglect (NCPCA, 1995; NCCAFV, 1999; Perry, 2000). Thus, about 47 out of every 1000 children are victims of child maltreatment.

No single cause exists for parental abuse and/or neglect (i.e., maltreatment) of a child. Rather, many different factors influence the relationship between the parent and his or her child. Such factors include individual family member characteristics, the psychosocial environment of the family (Campbell, 1997; Corse, Schmid, & Trickett, 1990; DePanfilis, 1996), and the stressors upon or limited support system available to the family within a broader community context (Bronfenbrenner; Cicchetti & Rizley, as cited in Brady, Posner, Lang, & Rosati, 1994; Polansky, Ammons, & Gaudin, 1985).

Whether abuse occurs in a family is not bound by socioeconomic level. Actually, parental abuse and neglect occur across all socioeconomic levels. Limited resources and support systems, and increased stress due to poverty, however, may contribute to the likelihood of child maltreatment (Barnett, Vondra, & Shonk, 1996; Kotch, Browne, Ringwalt, & Stewart, 1995; Levine as cited in Brady et al., 1994). Parental history of abuse/neglect (Chiancone, 1997; Egeland, 1993; Growenstein & Spunt, 1997; Guterman, 1997; Kaplan-Sanoff, 1996; Littey, Kowalski, & Minor, 1996; Perloff & Buckner, 1996) and presence of domestic violence (Aron & Olson, 1997; Dystra & Alop, 1996; Kaplan, 1996) are other factors with potential links to child abuse and neglect.

Beyond limited resources, increased stress, and parental history of abuse, other factors, such as parental abuse of alcohol and other drugs, have been implicated in child maltreatment (Brady et al., 1994; Carten,

1996; Crimmins, Langley, Brownstein, & Spunt, 1997; Gaudin, 1993; Guterman, 1997; Rose, 1991; Wright, Garrison, Wright, & Stimmel, 1991). More and more children each year experience trauma by having been prenatally exposed to alcohol and other drugs such as marijuana and cocaine (Chasnoff, Anson, Hatcher, Stenson, Iaukea, & Randolph, 1998; Madison, Johnson, Seikel, Arnold, & Schultheis, 1998; NCPCA, 1995, Streissguth, 1999). Although prevalence data vary, it has been estimated by the National Institute on Drug Abuse (NIDA) that approximately 221,000 children are born prenatally exposed to illegal drugs and for 45,000 of those children the drug exposure is to cocaine (Chasnoff et al., 1998). The primary illegal drugs to which infants are exposed in utero include cocaine and marijuana. Generally, newborns are prenatally exposed to cocaine at a rate of approximately 1-4.5% and to marijuana at a rate of approximately 3-20%, which suggests that marijuana is used more widely than cocaine (Gomby & Shiono, 1991). Prenatal exposure to the drug alcohol, however, surpasses the use of the illegal drugs (Brady et al., 1994). The Centers for Disease Control and Prevention (as cited by the National Organization on Fetal Alcohol Syndrome, 1999) reported that in 1993, there were 6.7 babies born with Fetal Alcohol Syndrome (FAS) for every 10,000 births. In 1996 it was reported that the rate of babies born affected by prenatal exposure to alcohol was 19.5 per 10,000 live births with estimates as high as 30 per 10,000 live births (National Organization of Fetal Alcohol Syndrome, 1999).

IMPACT OF TRAUMA ON DEVELOPMENTAL AND EDUCATIONAL OUTCOMES

Child trauma, such as abuse, neglect, and prenatal exposure to alcohol and other drugs, negatively impacts children in a myriad of ways. There are overlapping effects of experiencing abuse, neglect, and exposure to alcohol or other drugs in utero. The relationship between these traumatic experiences and developmental and educational outcomes are only in the beginning stages of exploration (Chasnoff et al., 1998). It is, therefore, difficult to predict which type of abuse affects which type of domain: behavioral, developmental and/or academic. Some research has shown, however, that experiences with or exposure to these types of traumas negatively affects child development, emotional well-being, and subsequently negatively affects child educational outcomes (Dore, 1999; English, 1998; Perry, 1997; Perry, 1999; Turpin, Tarico, Low, Jemelka, & McClellan, 1993).

Impact of Trauma on Child Development

The effects of child maltreatment and prenatal exposure to alcohol and drugs last throughout life. These effects negatively impact human development from infancy through childhood, adolescence, and adulthood. Child development domains affected include: physical, cognitive, sensory, and motor; behavior and emotional; and communication, including language and literacy acquisition.

Children affected by traumatic experiences, such as abuse and/or neglect, after birth are more likely also to have experienced premature births, low birth-weight, disorganized behavioral states and birth defects (Brady et al., 1994; Chasnoff et al., 1998). Premature births prevent the fetus from growing fully in utero placing the child at increased risk for medical and developmental problems, as well as for learning and behavioral problems (Chasnoff et al., 1998). Disorganized behavioral states may be marked by feeding problems, sleep disturbances, extreme irritability and over-sensitivity to touch, movement or eye contact (Griffith as cited in Chasnoff et al., 1998). Moreover, prenatal exposure to alcohol can lead to Fetal Alcohol Syndrome (FAS) or Alcohol-Related Birth Defects (ARBD). Consequences of FAS or ARBD can include central nervous system damage resulting in developmental and cognitive delays, small head circumferences, and abnormal facial feature developments (Rosett, 1980). Small head circumference, in turn, is suggestive of poor brain growth, which makes it a significant indicator of being at risk for poor developmental outcome (Chasnoff et al., 1998). Facial abnormalities include a small head circumference, narrow eyes, flat and long filtrum or upper lip, and a flattened nose bridge (Rosett, 1980; Streissguth, 1999).

Behavior problems can appear as a result of exposure or experience with trauma. Such behavioral problems include overactive or reduced reflexes, poor coordination or motor control; limited visual or auditory orientation to stimuli; and limited abilities to regulate one's states (Brady et al., 1994; Chasnoff et al., 1998, Streissguth, 1999). As an infant, motor difficulties include reduced skills in reaching, grabbing, and exploring objects. There also may be indications of overactive or reduced reflexes and limited coordination of sucking and swallowing responses. Infants and children exposed to trauma have difficulty regulating their own states. For example, infants may cry uncontrollably for no apparent reason without being able to be comforted. Infants also may go into a deep unresponsive sleep (Chasnoff et al., 1998). Children also have been found to exhibit low developmental scores and disorganized play skills. For example, children exposed to alcohol in utero were found to engage in stacking and knocking down toys rather than engaging in systematic, symbolic or functional play (Fried & Watkinson, 1990). The National Association for Families and Addiction Research and Education (NAFARE) conducted a longitudinal study of school-age children who were prenatally exposed to drugs such as cocaine and alcohol (as cited in Chasnoff et al., 1998, pp. 10-16). NAFARE found behaviors to occur such as depression, social problems, and aggressive behavior (Table 1).

Additionally, these children experience insecure attachment with caretakers, which includes difficulty bonding and negative effects on future relationships. Attachment problems manifest as being either too friendly or affectionate or being too independent, as demonstrated by rarely seeking help or comfort from an adult (Ainsworth, 1978). Difficulties with attachment to caregivers can interrupt learning and social development skills (Levy & Orlans, 1998).

Communication skills also are found to be depressed in children who have been exposed to trauma such as abuse, neglect, and prenatal exposure to alcohol and other drugs (Mentis, 1998). Such communication problems may include increased articulatory or phonological problems (Madison, Johnson, Seikel, Arnold, & Schultheis, 1998), disorganized thinking, limited vocabulary skills (Bland-Stewart, Seymour, Beeghly, & Frank, 1998), low comprehension and expressive language skills, and difficulty acquiring academic or print literacy. Mentis and Lundgren (1995) found that children prenatally exposed to cocaine exhibited problems in clearly connecting conversational topics and utilized more immature syntactic structures than their non-exposed counterparts. Communication delays/disorders may be a result of reduced frequency and quality of social interactions or the result of neurological changes resulting from abuse and neglect (Perry as cited in Westby, 1999).

The Impact of Trauma on Educational Outcomes

All children who enter school bring with them a wide range of behaviors. For the children who have been traumatized or prenatally exposed to alcohol or other drugs, the behaviors that they bring are often difficult to manage or understand in the educational setting. Teachers are often unprepared for children with these types of histories/experiences, who often do not respond to typical educational strategies or teaching methods. Teachers or uninformed caregivers may see the behavior of these children as willfully disobedient rather than an inability to regulate

TABLE 1. Types and Descriptions of Behaviors Exhibited by Traumatized Children

Type of Behavior	Description of Behavior
Anxiety/Depression	Feels need to be perfect; feels unloved; feels others out to get him; feels worthless or inferior; nervous/high-strung/tense; sad/unhappy; worries; nervous/anxious.
Social Problems	Acts too young for age; clingy; does not get along with others; gets teased a lot; not liked by other children.
Thought Problems	Cannot get mind off of certain thoughts; repeats certain acts over and again; stares; strange ideas; strange behavior.
Attention Problems	Cannot concentrate for long; cannot sit still/restless; confused; daydreams; impulsive; poor schoolwork.
Delinquent Problems	No guilt after misbehaving; lies/cheats; prefers older kids; steals; hangs around with kids who get into trouble.
Aggressive Problems	Argues a lot; demands attention; destroys things of his own or others; disobedient at home and/or at school; sudden changes in mood; talks too much; unusually loud; temper tantrums.

From NAFARE as cited in Chasnoff et al., 1998, pg. 13-14.

one's own states (Chasnoff, 2000). This belief sets up a paradigm of lower expectations for those "problem" children. Gunter and Denny (cited in Audet & Tankersly, 1998) reported that teachers typically do not implement behavior strategies that have been shown to be successful for changing behaviors, but more frequently rely on the "efficient" use of verbal directives to manage behavior. The over-reliance on verbal directions may increase the use of punitive and disapproving measures for children (Audet & Tankersly, 1998) with emotional and behavioral difficulties resulting from traumatic experiences.

RESULTS OF A NEEDS SURVEY

Two surveys (March 1998 and January 2000) were conducted to determine the community's perceived need for a comprehensive assessment center (see Appendix A for surveys). The potential responses to the need for a trauma assessment center ranged from "no need" to "significant need." In 1998, surveys were sent to a total of 396 human service professionals in eight southwestern Michigan counties. Of the 396 distributed surveys, 230 (58%) were returned. Of these returned surveys,

87% indicated a "strong" to "significant need." In 2000, the survey was again distributed to 50 more human service professionals, which yielded a return rate of 52% (27 returned surveys). Eighty percent of the respondents indicated a "strong" to "significant need" for a comprehensive developmental assessment center to serve traumatized children.

CTAC officially opened in March 2000 and has consistently received a large number of referrals from numerous child welfare agencies, which confirms the need for a trauma assessment center. Currently, the CTAC team conducts comprehensive assessments two afternoons per week, for six children (3 per afternoon) per week. Since opening, there have been no assessment vacancies and we are currently maintaining a 4-5 week waiting list.

DEVELOPMENT OF A CHILDREN'S TRAUMA ASSESSMENT CENTER

CTAC was conceptualized in 1998 and established with in-kind support from Western Michigan University (WMU), and with funding from the Kalamazoo and Fetzer Foundations in the year of 1999. The center director, James Henry, PhD, Social Work, assembled faculty and staff from WMU who were all part of the same college (The College of Health and Human Services) and from the southwestern Michigan community. In addition to Dr. Henry, the current core CTAC staff includes Ben Atchison, PhD, Occupational Therapy; Constance Black-Pond, MA, Social Work/Counseling; Yvette D. Hyter, PhD, CCC, Speech-Language Pathology; and Mark Sloane, DO, Pediatrics. A child traumatized by abuse, neglect, and prenatal exposure to alcohol is affected in many developmental areas; therefore, it was important to assemble a team of professionals that would be able to simultaneously address some of those issues. In addition to the currently represented disciplines, input from the disciplines of educational psychology, nursing, and nutrition would be important additions. Additionally, from each discipline there are at least two undergraduate or graduate student clinicians completing their clinical practicum through a CTAC placement.

The CTAC team met weekly from December 1999 through February 2000 to develop the trauma center assessment protocol and to facilitate its implementation. In January, upon the return and analysis of the needs survey, announcements were sent to the social service agencies in southwestern Michigan, which were followed-up with presentations and a question-answer session for social service professionals in the region. The doors of CTAC were opened in March 2000; this was commemorated with an open house.

CTAC: A Model of Family Centered and Transdisciplinary Practices

Two concepts that provide support for CTAC are encoded in federal policy in the Individuals with Disabilities Education Act (IDEA, U. S. Congress, 1997). These concepts include family centered practices and a transdisciplinary model of collaborative assessment and intervention.

Family Centered Practices. Family centered practices indicate that the needs, strengths, and priorities of the families drive the assessment and intervention process (Crais & Wilson, 1996). This process involves family members (caretakers) as essential members of the assessment and/or intervention team. Also, this practice helps caretakers to identify concerns, priorities, and resources for their child (Crais, 1991; Donahue-Kilburg, 1993). Family centered practices emerge from Bronfenbrenner's (1979) Ecological Theory and from Family Systems Theory (Becvar & Becvar as cited in Hammer, 1998; Nelson, 1998). Ecological Theory emphasizes the importance of considering the context in which the behaviors in question occur. Similarly, one assumption of the Family Systems Theory is that the child is part of a system, a family system, that includes individual but interdependent members; therefore, the child can only be understood in the context of this system or in the context of the relationships that form the family with which the child resides. Also, there are three other assumptions of the Family Systems Theory. The second is that patterns of behavior exhibited by one member (i.e., the child) can influence the other members and vice versa. Third, families go through changes (e.g., divorce, or in the case of foster children the removal or addition of another foster child) that can positively or negatively influence the relationships within the family. Fourth, each member of the family has a different perspective of the relationships that exist in his or her particular family system. For example, Hammer (1998) states that " . . . communicating, behaving and failing to act or communicate are in themselves forms of communication, and although a person may ascribe meaning to another person's behavior, that meaning may only be true for the person doing the ascribing" (p. 6).

To implement family centered practices and to understand the family system, information must be gathered from the family members. This information is best gathered using an ethnographic interviewing method (Hammer, 1998; Hyter, 2000; Westby, 1990). The objective of ethnography is to understand a worldview from perspectives that are different from one's own, and which will help to understand how other people perceive their own lives (Spradley, 1979). Ethnographic interviewing involves conversing with the family using open-ended interviews to gain access to the perspectives of the family members (Spradley, 1979). A complete and accurate understanding of the family's perspective will permit collaborative identification and development of intervention strategies that are aligned with existing family values and practices (Hyter, 2000), yielding higher compliance with intervention strategies.

Collaboration Through a Transdisciplinary Service Model. Collaboration is the practice of multiple disciplines (and caretakers) collectively identifying and defining mutual problems, and then cooperatively generating solutions to those problems (DiMeo, Merritt, & Culatta, 1998; Hyter & Self, 1999; Idol, Paolucci-Whitcomb, & Nevin, 1986; McCormick & Schiefelbusch, 1990). For this project, collaborative services are delivered through a transdisciplinary model.

Within a transdisciplinary model, all team members share responsibility for child outcomes by expanding and exchanging knowledge with other team members (Linder, 1993; Prelock, Miller, & Reed, 1995). A transdisciplinary model includes the team processes of joint functioning, continuous staff development, and role release (Woodruff & McGonigel as cited in Prelock et al., 1995). Joint functioning consists of all team members performing required service delivery functions together whenever possible; that is, all team members primarily will complete assessments, plan intervention, and carry out intervention activities together when possible (McCormick & Schiefelbusch, 1990). Continuous staff development (McCormick & Schiefelbusch, 1990) occurs when team members train and receive training from each other, and includes concepts such as role extension, enrichment, expansion, and exchange (Woodruff & McGonigel as cited in Prelock et al., 1995). Role extension and enrichment refer to team members increasing their knowledge about their own discipline and about the other disciplines with which they are working. Role expansion and exchange occur when team members directly share information with each other regarding terminology and procedures (Prelock et al., 1995). Role release refers to team members sharing information and skill functions (Linder, 1993; McCormick & Schiefelbusch, 1990); that is, team members take on one another's roles. For example, during an evaluation at CTAC, the occupational therapist may evaluate a child's hand manipulation skills and strength as the child handles the objects he or she has requested. At the same time, the speech-language pathologist may evaluate a child's communicative functions (e.g., the purposes for communicating such as to request an object or action). Through role release, the occupational therapist learns from the speech-language pathologist information about and techniques for assessing or recognizing communicative functions. Similarly, the speech-language pathologist learns from the occupational therapist information about and techniques for assessing hand manipulation skills and hand strength. Later, members of both professions will be able to utilize the knowledge and skills learned from the other profession in their respective future assessments.

Foley (1990) describes four principles that underlie the theoretical rationale for using the transdisciplinary model. First, developmental problems typically result from an accumulation of events rather than a single event. Second, crossover effects may occur with developmental problems producing a negative impact on multiple developmental domains. Third, systematic analyses are required to understand complex problems. A traumatized child is affected in numerous developmental areas including cognitive, neurological, language and literacy, behavioral, socio-emotional and physical; therefore, when multiple issues simultaneously occur, the symptoms are complex and require complex and multi-layered solutions. Fourth, children do not develop in a vacuum and their development, or lack thereof, should be considered in the context of their environment. Consequently, the assessment and intervention must consider the interaction between familial, societal, and individual factors to determine the depth and range of potential risk, and to determine the best solutions to reduce or address that risk (Hummel & Prizant, 1993; Nelson, 1998).

CTAC: Putting Theory into Practice

Collaboration through a transdisciplinary model and family centered practices are put into practice at CTAC. CTAC is designed to maximize developmental and educational outcomes of children who have been traumatized by abuse, neglect, and exposure to alcohol and other drugs by (1) conducting comprehensive transdisciplinary and family focuses assessments, (2) providing recommendations for the child's care that will facilitate positive developmental and educational outcomes, (3) providing caretaker support, and (4) advocating for appropriate educational service provisions for the child and his or her family (biological or foster).

Currently, CTAC completes comprehensive transdisciplinary assessments on approximately 300 children per year (averaging six children per week, three children per day–Monday and Friday afternoons) who have been referred for services primarily by child welfare agencies. Assessments include a medical examination and assessments of cognitive/academic, language/literacy, physical, emotional/behavioral, social/familial skills and level of trauma. The assessments are followed by a comprehensive and detailed report (see Appendix B for sample report format) which is discussed with the child's caretakers and forwarded to the referring party–the social service agencies. The CTAC process is depicted in a flow-chart presented in Figure 1. The assessment protocol is presented in Table 2.

Each assessment lasts approximately 2-3 hours within a one-day period; however, the assessment can be completed over two days if the length of the assessment is too long for a particular child. In addition to developmental assessments CTAC also conducts Fetal Alcohol Syndrome/Fetal Alcohol Effects assessments and diagnoses. In July 2000, the CTAC staff received training at the Chicago Research Triangle from a multidisciplinary team under the direction of Dr. Ira Chasnoff, an international expert in the diagnosis and treatment of prenatal drug exposure. CTAC is the only transdisciplinary team in southwestern Michigan trained to provide FAS/FAE diagnosis.

FUTURE CTAC GOALS

Conceptualizing, planning, developing, and implementing CTAC required two years (i.e., from 1998-2000). The first year focused on conceptualizing the center. The second year focused on acquiring support, resources, staff, and protocols for the center. After one year of operation (2000-2001), the CTAC team has realized that there is a significant need to inform caretakers and educators about the effects of trauma on child development across all domains. Without such knowledge, adults frequently mislabel and misunderstand the actions of these children, which further stigmatizes and isolates them. It is important to help care-

FIGURE 1. Southwestern Michigan Children's Trauma Assessment Center (CTAC) Assessment Flow Chart

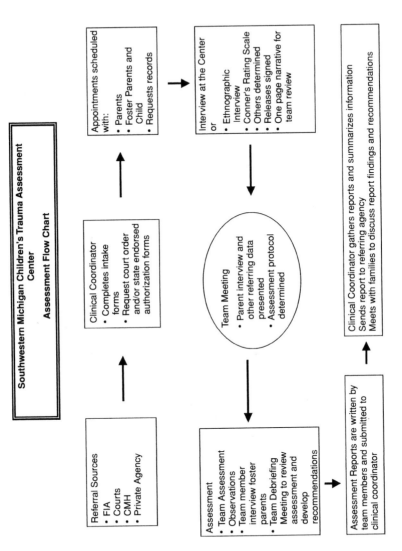

Southwestern Michigan Children's Trauma Assessment
Center

Assessment Flow Chart

Referral Sources
• FIA
• Courts
• CMH
• Private Agency

Clinical Coordinator
• Completes intake forms
• Request court order and/or state endorsed authorization forms

Appointments scheduled with:
• Parents
• Foster Parents and Child
• Requests records

Interview at the Center or
• Ethnographic Interview
• Conner's Rating Scale
• Others determined
• Releases signed
• One page narrative for team review

Team Meeting
• Parent interview and other referring data presented
• Assessment protocol determined

Assessment
• Team Assessment
• Observations
• Team member interview foster parents
• Team Debriefing Meeting to review assessment and develop recommendations

Assessment Reports are written by team members and submitted to clinical coordinator

Clinical Coordinator gathers reports and summarizes information
Sends report to referring agency
Meets with families to discuss report findings and recommendations

TABLE 2. The CTAC Assessment Protocol[1]

Hawaii Early Learning Profile (HELP)
The HELP is a comprehensive developmental assessment, which includes 685 criterion-referenced items covering six developmental domains. These domains include cognition, language, gross motor, fine motor, social-emotional, and self-help. Items have excellent construct validity against other well-known scales and standardized tests.

The Kaufman Brief Intelligence Test (K-BIT)
The K-BIT is a standardized test, which measures verbal and nonverbal intelligence appropriate for ages 4-90. There are two subtests; Vocabulary, which measures verbal intelligence and Matrices, which evaluates nonverbal intelligence. Reliability for test retest and split-half measures are strong as is validity determined by concurrent analysis.

The Pediatric Early Elementary Examination (PEEX)
The PEEX-2 is a comprehensive, criterion-referenced assessment designed to tap function in the fine motor, graphomotor, receptive and expressive language, gross-motor, visual and auditory memory, sequential processing, visual processing, and attention.

The Pediatric Examination of Educational Readiness at Middle Childhood (PEERMID)
The PEERMID is similar to the PEEX in terms of items, administration and scoring. The PEERMID measures the same developmental parameters as the PEEX, in addition, higher cognition.

Test of Early Reading Abilities–Second Edition (TERA-2)
The TERA-2 is a standardized norm-referenced instrument designed to measure the reading ability of young children. This test contains items that measure knowledge of contextual meaning, alphabet, and literacy conventions.

Gray Oral Reading Test (GORT-3)
The GORT-3 is a standardized, norm-referenced instrument, which measures oral reading in school-age children and adolescents, and helps to diagnose oral reading difficulties.

Test of Written Language (TOWL)
The TOWL provides a measure of writing competence through spontaneous and contrived formats. It includes several subtests focusing on spelling conventions; vocabulary, syntax, and grammar; character and plot development and compositional skills; word usage; spelling ability; use of punctuation; and simple and complex sentence construction.

Reactive Attachment Disorder Questionnaire (RADQ)
Conner's Revised Parent Rating Scale for Parents/ for Teachers
The Connor's is a comprehensive behavioral rating scale that is designed for children ages 3-17 and used both for screening and monitoring of progress. A set of sub-scales assesses the child for oppositional defiance, inattentiveness, hyperactivity, anxious/extreme shyness, perfectionism, and social problems.

Draw a Person Test (DAP)
DAP is a drawing technique for social emotional assessment of children. Scoring is non-standardized and is completed in conjunction with a narrative summary about the picture.

Parent Trauma Symptom Intake Questionnaire
This self-report assessment for children between 3-6 years of age identifies critical behaviors indicative of child trauma that the child exhibits pre and post trauma.

Traumagenic Impact of Maltreatment Rating Scale
This is a checklist designed to provide a brief summary of nine major traumagenic areas associated with child maltreatment. These areas include traumatic sexualization, eroticization, betrayal and loss, stigmatization, powerlessness, self-blaming, destructive acting out, loss of body integrity, development of dissociative disorder, and development of attachment disorder.

Child Trauma Safety Checklist
This is a self-report of a child's perception of safe context for which a rating is applied from "safe" to "very dangerous" using a graphic expression of a smiling to sad face to enable the younger child to respond.

Trauma Symptom Checklist for Children
This self-assessment is designed to screen for post trauma symptoms across several clinical sub-scales of social emotional behavior. These include anxiety, depression, anger, posttraumatic stress, dissociation, fantasy, sexual concerns, sexual preoccupation, and sexual distress.

Children's Depression Inventory
This is a 27-item self-report of depressive symptomatology used with school-age children and adolescents.

This list of assessment instruments was gathered from Atchison, B. (2000). Southwest Michigan Child Trauma Assessment Center: Student information manual. Western Michigan University, Unpublished document.

¹Note that not all assessments are administered to all children. The assessment protocol is developed per each child based on his or her specific needs as identified through the ethnographic interview of caretakers and teachers.

givers and educators develop strategies that will help to increase positive educational outcomes for these children, as they frequently do not respond to traditional school structure and discipline techniques. Several educators have reported to CTAC staff that they have tried many strategies with the traumatized child in their care, and that they are looking for new and more appropriate solutions to meet the child's needs. Additionally, CTAC staff have realized that a period of ongoing support is necessary to provide to caretakers and educators caring for and educating traumatized children an opportunity to expand their knowledge to create alternative responses to these children. The goal is to enhance positive classroom management and to optimize the children's learning potential. Moreover, it has become evident that a significant communication and collaboration gap exists between caretakers, educators, and social service workers working with children traumatized by abuse, neglect, and/or prenatal exposure to alcohol.

To implement these goals, there is a need to hire additional staff. In November 2000, we received a grant that will support a home interventionist for the year 2001-2002. The interventionist will provide specific support to caregivers regarding the impact of trauma on child development. Also, with caregivers, the interventionist will jointly develop strategies which consider the unique characteristics of the child that will help support the child in the home. Strategies will include altering the existing environment, and home management strategies. In addition to the interventionist, we are hoping to expand the core transdisciplinary team to include a nurse and an educational psychologist to assist with assessments and facilitate interactions between CTAC and the school systems.

Another goal of CTAC is to interface more frequently with the educational system to offer support and information. Currently, CTAC staff members have been involved in some Individual Education Plan Committee (IEPC) meetings. There is a need, however, for more consistent involvement in these meetings as a way to support educators' understanding of the relationship between the child's experienced trauma (i.e., abuse and/or neglect or prenatal exposure to alcohol) and behavior. Also, participation in IEPC meetings serves to inform the educational system on the type of assessments and treatment recommendations that CTAC can provide. It is important to develop educator empathy. Often these children are viewed as being willfully disobedient, but due to sensory processing regulatory disorders resulting from the experienced trauma, the children often are unable to manage or control their own behaviors. Chasnoff et al. (1998) suggest that the ability to be empathic is the most important aspect to responding to various behaviors exhibited by traumatized children.

Another future goal of CTAC is to provide a developmental enrichment program that will be designed to strengthen the participant's sensory processing skills, as well as language and literacy skills. The purpose of the enrichment program would be to provide short-term, but focused collaborative intervention for sensory processing problems that result in regulatory difficulties, and language and literacy difficulties. Through this enrichment program, CTAC staff and participating students will inform caretakers and educators about particular sensory processing problems and instruct them in techniques to use for improvement of particular problems. Also, caregivers will receive support for expanding the ways in which emergent and early literacy skills are facilitated.

CONCLUSIONS

Within the last year, CTAC staff members have:

- Developed and implemented a transdisciplinary team model that optimizes the use of professional expertise while minimizing the child's multiple interactions with professionals.
- Provided comprehensive assessments that include a medical examination, developmental, cognitive/academic, emotional/behavioral, social/familial, and trauma assessment for over 170 children.

- Conducted Fetal Alcohol Syndrome/Fetal Alcohol Effects assessments and diagnoses.
- Met with many caretakers regarding assessment results and recommendations for children's care.
- Attended several IEPC school meetings to advocate for the educational needs of children who were assessed by CTAC. It should be noted, however, that a potential long-term effect of advocating for the educational needs of the CTAC participants, is that the needs of all students will be better served.
- Testified in Family Court to represent the best interest of children.
- Developed an in-home pilot program with caretakers that focuses on supporting caretakers in developing and implementing activities that can be carried out in the home of the children. Following each assessment, the CTAC team makes recommendations for intervention if required, further assessments, or for the implementation of activities that can be carried out in the home. In-home recommendations focus on speech-language, social emotional, and state regulation issues (i.e., a group of behaviors that typically occur together such as bodily activity, breathing patterns and physiological responses to external stimuli [Paul, 1995]). Some strategies that have been implemented focus on helping families (1) identify factors (e.g., medical difficulties, learning problems, emotional issues, low thresholds for frustrations, heightened sensitivity to external stimuli) that may contribute to the child's difficulties, (2) identify "new" behaviors to replace the difficult behaviors, (3) work with the interventionist to jointly identify approaches (interventions) to address the difficulties of the child, and (4) implement such techniques as modeling and role play. Further, such interventions may include making changes to the home environment and management techniques (Chasnoff et al., 1998).
- Provided four workshops at the state and national level regarding the CTAC program. The workshops focused on the effect that abuse, neglect, and prenatal exposure to alcohol have on the developmental outcomes of children. These workshops also included information on the conceptualization of CTAC, the transdisciplinary team assessment process, and presented case histories to demonstrate the developmental, psychosocial, and FAS assessments that are conducted.

CTAC staff members have accomplished a great deal during the first year of service; however, we have many other goals to accomplish through our program. For example, there is a need to establish a consistent line of funding for the operation of the clinic. Additionally, there are plans to develop and implement effective strategies to teach and support educators and parents regarding developmental issues related to child maltreatment and the management of traumatized children.

REFERENCES

Avery, R. J. (1999). Identifying obstacles to adoption in New York State's out of home care system. *Child Welfare, 78* (5), 653-671.

Barnett, D., Vondra, J. I., Shonk, & S.M. (1996). Self perceptions, motivation, and school functioning of low-income maltreated and comparison children. *Child Abuse and Neglect, 20* (5), 397-410.

Bland-Stewart, L. M., Seymour, H. N., Beeghly, M., & Frank, D. A. (1998). Semantic development of African-American children prenatally exposed to cocaine. *Seminars in Speech and Language, 19* (2), 167-187.

Brady, J. P., Posner, M., Lang, C., & Rosati, M. J. (1994). *Risk and reality: The implications of prenatal exposure to alcohol and other drugs.* Available from *http://www. evalustats.com/drugkids.htm*

Brofenbrenner, U. (1979). *Ecology of human development.* Cambridge, MA: Harvard University Press.

Campbell, L. (1997). Child neglect and intensive-family-preservation practice. *Families in Society, 78* (3), 280-290.

Carten, A. J. (1996). Rebuilding families in the aftermath of addiction. *Social Work, 41* (2), 214-223.

Chasnoff, I. J. (2000). Presentation at Fetal Alcohol Training Seminar. Chicago Research Triangle, Chicago, IL.

Chasnoff, I. J., Anson, A., Hatcher, R., Stenson, H., Iaukea, K., & Randolph, L. A. (1998). Prenatal exposure to cocaine and other drugs: Outcome at four to six years. *Annals of New York Academy of Sciences, 846,* 314-328.

Chiancone, J. (1997). Troubled family legacies and resilience. *ABA Child Law Practice, 16* (2), 24-29.

Corse, S. J., Schmid, K., & Trickett, P. K. (1990). Social network characteristics of mothers in abusing and nonabusing families and their relationships to parenting beliefs. *Journal of Community Psychology, 18,* 44-59.

Crais, E., & Wilson, L. (1996). The role of parents in child assessment: Self-evaluation by practicing professionals. *Infant-Toddler Intervention, 6,* 125-147.

Crimmins, S., Langley, S., Brownstein, H. H., & Spunt, B. J. (1997). Convicted women who have killed children: A self-psychology perspective. *Journal of Interpersonal Violence, 12* (1), 49-69.

Dale, G., Kendall, M., Humber, M., & Sheehan, L. (1999). Screening young foster children for posttraumatic stress disorder and responding to their needs for treatment. *The APSAC Advisor 12,* (2) 6-8.

DePanfilis, D. (1996). Social isolation of neglectful families: A review of social support assessment and intervention models. *Child Maltreatment, 1* (1) 37-52.

DiMeo, J. H., Merritt, D. D., & Culatta, B. (1998). Collaborative partnerships and decision making. In D. D. Merritt & B. Culatta (Eds.), *Language intervention in the classroom*. San Diego, CA: Singular Publishing Group, Inc.

Donahue-Kilburg, G. (1992). *Family-centered early intervention for communication disorders: Prevention and treatment*. Gaithersburg, MD: Aspen Publishers, Inc.

Dore, M. (1999). Emotionally and behaviorally disturbed children in the child welfare system: Points of preventive intervention. *Children and Youth Services Review, 21* (4) 7-29.

Egeland, B. (1993). A history of abuse is a major risk factor for abusing the next generation. In R. J. Gelles & D. R. Loseke (Eds.), *Current controversies on family violence* (pp. 197-208). Newbury Park, CA.

English, D. (1998). The extent and consequences of child maltreatment. *Future of Children,* Spring, 1999, 39-50.

Foley, G. M. (1990). Portrait of the arena evaluation: Assessment in the trans-disciplinary approach. In E. D. Gibs & D. M. Teti (Eds.), *Interdisciplinary assessment of infants*. Baltimore, MD: Paul H. Brookes.

Ford, J., Racusin, R., Ellis, C., Davis, W., Reiser, J., Fleischer, A., & Thomas, J. (2000). Child maltreatment, other trauma exposure, and posttraumatic symptomatology among children with oppositional defiant and attention deficit hyperactivity disorders. *Child Maltreatment, 5* (3), 205-217.

Fried, P. A., & Watkinson, B. (1990). 36- and 48-month neurobehavioral follow-up of children prenatally exposed to marijuana, cigarettes, and alcohol. *Developmental and Behavioral Pediatrics, 11* (2), 49-58.

Gaudin, J. M. (1993, April). *Child neglect: A guide for intervention*. Available from *http://www.calib.com/nccanch/pubs/usermanuals/neglect/index.htm*.

Gomby, D., & Shiono, P. (1991, Spring). Estimating the number of substance-exposed infants. *The Future of Children, 1* (1), 17-25.

Guterman, N. B. (1997). Parental violence towards children. In N. K. Phillips & S. L. A. Straussner (Eds.), *Children in the urban environment: Linking social policy and clinical practice*. (pp. 113-134). Springfield, IL: Charles C. Thomas, Pub.

Hammer, C. S. (1998). Toward a "thick description" of families: Using ethnography to overcome the obstacles to providing family-centered early intervention services. *American Journal of Speech-Language Pathology, 7* (1), 5-22.

Hummel, L. J., & Prizant, B. M. (1993). A socioemotional perspective for understanding social difficulties of school-age children with language disorders. *Language, Speech, and Hearing Services in Schools, 24,* 216-224.

Hyter, Y. D., & Self, T. (1998). Practical issues in communication therapy: Intervention for children with behavior and language disorders. In D. Rogers-Adkinson & P. Griffith (Eds.), *Communication disorders and children with psychiatric and behavioral disorders* (pp. 367-402). San Diego, CA: Singular Publishing Group, Inc.

Hyter, Y. D. (February 2000). Seeing purple: Using ethnographic research methods as a standard rather than the exception in clinical service delivery. Guest Editorial. *The ASHA Leader, 5* (3), 10.

Idol, L., Paolucci-Whitcomb, P., & Nevin, A. (1986). *Collaborative consultation*. Rockville, MD: Aspen.

Kaplan, S.J. (1996). *Family violence: A clinical and legal guide*. Washington, DC: American Psychiatric Press, Inc.

Kaplan-Sanoff, M. (1996). *The impact of maternal substance abuse on young children: Myths and realities.* Washington, DC: National Association of Social Workers.

Kotch, J. B., Browne, D. C., Ringwalt, C. L., Stewart, P.W. (1995). Risk of child abuse or neglect in a cohort of low-income children. *Child Abuse and Neglect, 19* (9), 1115-1130.

Levin, M. D. (1996). *Pediatric early elementary examination.* Cambridge, MA: Educators Publishing Service, Inc.

Levy, M., & Orlans, M. (1998). *Attachment, trauma, and healing.* Washington, DC: Child Welfare League of America.

Linder, T. (1993). *Transdisciplinary play-based intervention: Guidelines for developing a meaningful curriculum for young children.* Baltimore: Paul H. Brookes.

Litty, C. G., Kowalski, R., & Minor, S. (1996). Moderating effects of physical abuse and perceived social support on the potential to abuse. *Child Abuse and Neglect, 20* (4), 305-314.

Madison, C. L., Johnson, J. M., Seikel, J. A., Arnold, M., & Schultheis, L. (1998). Comparative study of the phonology of preschool children prenatally exposed to cocaine and multiple drugs and non-exposed children. *Journal of Communication Disorders, 31,* 231-244.

McCormick, L., & Schiefelbusch, R. L. (1990). *Early language intervention: An introduction (2nd ed.).* Columbus, OH: Merrill.

Mentis, M. (1998). In utero cocaine exposure and language development. *Seminars in Speech and Language, 19* (2), 147-165.

Mentis, M., & Lundgren, K. (1995). Effects of prenatal exposure to cocaine and associated risk factors on language development. *Journal of Speech and Hearing Research, 38,* 1303-1318.

Nash, M. R., Hulsey, T. L., Sexton, M. C., Harralson, T. L., & Lambert, W. (1993). Long term sequelae of childhood sexual abuse: Perceived family environment, psychopathology, and dissociation. *Journal of Consulting and Clinical Psychology, 61* (2), 276-283.

National Organization of Fetal Alcohol Syndrome (1999). *FAS community resource center.* Available from *http://www.come-over.to/FASCRC.*

National Committee to Prevent Child Abuse (1995, December). *Child abuse and neglect: Statistics from the National Committee to Prevent Child Abuse.* Available from *http://www.vix.com/men/abuse/studies/child-ma.html.*

National Council on Child Abuse & Family Violence (1999). *Child abuse information.* Available from *http://www.nccafv.org/child.htm.*

National Institute on Drug Abuse (NIDA) (1991). *National household survey on drug abuse.* Rockville, MD: Substance Abuse and Mental Health Service Administration.

Nelson, N. W. (1998). *Childhood language disorders in context: Infancy through adolescence.* (2nd edition). Boston, MA: Allyn & Bacon.

Paul, R. (1995). *Language disorders from infancy through adolescence: Assessment and intervention.* Boston, MA: Mosby.

Perloff, J. N., & Buckner, J. C. (1996). Fathers of children on welfare: The impact on child well-being. *American Journal of Orthopsychiatry, 66* (4), 557-571.

Perry, B. D. (1999a). Effects of traumatic events on children. *Interdisciplinary Education Series, 2* (3), 9-17.

Perry, B. D. (1999b, August). Helping traumatized children: A brief overview for caregivers. *Child Trauma Academy Parent and Caregiver Education Series, 1* (3), 1-18.

Perry, B. D. (2000). Trauma and terror in childhood: The neuropsychiatric impact of childhood trauma. In I. Schulz, S. Carella, & D. O. Brady (Eds.), *Handbook of psychological injuries: Evaluation, treatment, and compensable damages.* American Bar Association Publishing.

Polansky, M. A., Ammons, P. W., & Gaudin, J.M. (1985). Loneliness and isolation in child neglect. *Social Casework, 66* (1), 38-47.

Prelock, P. A., Miller, B. L., & Reed, N. L. (1995). Collaborative partnerships in a language in the classroom program. *Language, Speech, and Hearing Services in Schools, 26* (3), 286-292.

Rose, S. (1991, August). Acknowledging abuse backgrounds of intensive case management clients. *Community Mental Health Journal, 27* (4), 255-263.

Rosett, H. (1980). A clinical perspective of the fetal alcohol syndrome. *Alcoholism: Clinical and Experimental Research, 4,* 119-122.

Spradley, J. (1979). *Ethnographic interviewing.* New York: Holt, Rinehart & Winston.

Streissguth, A. (1999). *Fetal alcohol syndrome: A guide for families and communities.* Baltimore, MD: Brookes Publishing Company.

Terr, L. (1991). Childhood traumas: An outline and overview. *American Journal of Psychiatry, 148* (1), 10-20.

Turpin, E., Tarico, V., Low, B., Jemelka, R., & McClellan, J. (1993). Child on child protective service caseloads: Prevalence and nature of serious emotional disturbance. *Child Abuse & Neglect, 17,* 345-355.

U. S. Department of Health and Human Services (1990). Fetal alcohol syndrome and other effects of alcohol on pregnancy outcome. In *Seventh special report to the U. S. Congress on alcohol and health from the Secretary of Health and Human Services* (pp. 139-161). Rockville, MD: U. S. Department of Health and Human Services.

United States Congress (1995, December). *Education of individuals with disabilities. 20 U.S.C. Chapter 33, Subchapter I–General Provisions.* Available from *http://www.lrp.com/ed/freelib/free-stats/u20-1409.htm*

Westby, C.E. (1990). Ethnographic interviewing: Asking the right questions to the right people in the right ways. *Journal of Childhood Communication Disorders, 13,* 101-111.

Westby, C. E. (1999). Assessment of pragmatic competence in children with psychiatric disorders. In D. Rogers-Adkinson & P. Griffith (Eds.), *Communication disorders and children with psychiatric and behavioral disorders* (pp. 177-258). San Diego, CA: Singular Publishing.

Wright, L. S., Garrison, J., Wright, N. B., & Stimmel, D. (1991). Childhood unhappiness and family stressors recalled by adult children of substance abusers. *Alcoholism Treatment Quarterly, 8* (4), 67-80.

Young, M. A. (1993). Tailoring services to child victims. *Technical Report,* 12 pp.

APPENDIX A
Needs Survey
March 1998

What is the need for developmental assessments that include physical, behavioral, psychological, educational, and trauma assessments for abused/neglected children that enter foster care or remain in their own home?

0	1	2	3	4	5
Don't Know	No Need		Some Need	Strong Need	Significant Need

If you are working with abused/neglected children would you refer children to such an assessment center?
Yes   No

If so approximately how many children per year could you refer? _____

What is the need for developmental assessments that include physical, behavioral, psychological, educational, and trauma assessments for children traumatized other than in abuse/neglect?

0	1	2	3	4	5
Don't Know	No Need		Some Need	Strong Need	Significant Need

If you are working with traumatized children would you refer children to such an assessment center?
Yes   No

If so approximately how many children per year could you refer? _____

What is the need for a treatment center that includes art therapy, music therapy, drama, dance, and massage along with clinical interventions to treat abused/neglected and traumatized children?

0	1	2	3	4	5
Don't Know	No Need		Some Need	Strong Need	Significant Need

Would you refer children to such a treatment center?
Yes   No

If so approximately how many children per year could you refer? _____

What is the need for a crisis-housing center that accommodates children (abused/neglected, mental health issues, and pre-delinquent) for temporary placements for assessment and stabilization for up to 90 days?

0	1	2	3	4	5
Don't Know	No Need		Some Need	Strong Need	Significant Need

Would you refer children for crisis housing?
Yes   No

If so approximately how many children per year could you refer? _____

APPENDIX A (continued)
January 2000
Trauma Center Survey Questions

1) What is the need for a trauma assessment center in southwestern Michigan to conduct multidisciplinary assessments of abused/neglected and other potentially traumatized children?

No need   Some need   Strong need   Very strong need

2) If such a trauma assessment center were available would you refer children to the center?

Yes   No

3) Approximately how many children could you refer to the trauma assessment during an average intake month? _____

Thank you for your cooperation. Please return as soon as possible.

APPENDIX B
Assessment Report
Ages 0-6

Child's Name:
Child's DOB:
Parent's Name:
Date Assessed:
Date of Report:
Referring agency and person:
Assessed by:
Reason for referral:
Overview of Assessment:

	Strengths	Within Age Expectations	Moderate Concern	Significant Concern
Physical/Medical				
Developmental				
Cognitive/Academic				
Social/Family				
Emotional/Behavioral				
Trauma Index				

APPENDIX B (continued)

Specific Domains:
I. Physical/Medical

	Normal	Concern
Height		
Weight		
Blood Pressure		
Hearing		
Vision		

Comments:

II. Developmental
Hawaii Early Learning Profile

Cognitive	
Language	
Gross Motor	
Fine Motor	
Social Emotional	
Self Help	

Comments:

Fetal Alcohol Syndrome Symptomology:

Overall Developmental:

Concerns	Strengths

III. Cognitive/Academic
Kaufman Brief Intelligence Test:

	IQ	Percentile
Vocabulary		
Matrices		
Composite		

Preschool/School Performance:

Comments:

Overall Cognitive/Academic

Concerns	Strengths

IV. Social/Family

Parent Perception of Child Interaction

Foster Parent Perception of Child Interaction

V. Emotional/Behavioral
Conner's Revised Parent Rating Scale: (completed by parent)

	T-Score	Clinically Significant
Oppositional		
Cognitive Problems/Inattention		
Hyperactivity		
Anxious-Shy		
Perfectionism		
Social Problems		

APPENDIX B (continued)

Psychosomatic		
Conner's ADHD Index		
Conner's Global Index: Restless-Impulsive		
Conner's Global Index: Emotional Lability		
Conner's Global Index: Total		
DSM-IV: Inattentive		
DSM-IV: Hyperactive-Impulsive		
DSM-IV Total		

Conner's Revised Parent Rating Scale: (completed by foster parent)

	T-Score	Clinically Significant
Oppositional		
Cognitive Problems/Inattention		
Hyperactivity		
Anxious-Shy		
Perfectionism		
Social Problems		
Psychosomatic		
Conner's ADHD Index		
Conner's Global Index: Restless-Impulsive		
Conner's Global Index: Emotional Lability		
Conner's Global Index: Total		
DSM-IV: Inattentive		
DSM-IV: Hyperactive-Impulsive		
DSM-IV Total		

Conner's Revised Parent Rating Scale: (completed by teacher)

	T-Score	Clinically Significant
Oppositional		
Cognitive Problems/Inattention		
Hyperactivity		
Anxious-Shy		
Perfectionism		
Social Problems		
Psychosomatic		
Conner's ADHD Index		
Conner's Global Index: Restless-Impulsive		

Conner's Global Index: Emotional Lability		
Conner's Global Index: Total		
DSM-IV: Inattentive		
DSM-IV: Hyperactive-Impulsive		
DSM-IV Total		

Comments:

Draw a Person:

Comments:

Overall Emotional/Behavioral:

Concerns	Strengths

VI. Trauma
Parent Trauma Symptom Intake Questionnaire:

	Asymptomatic	Symptomatic
Before Trauma		
After Trauma		

Comments:

Child Trauma Safety Checklist

Comments:

APPENDIX B (continued)

Traumagenic Impact of Maltreatment Rating Scale

Comments:	Absent-Severe 1 10	
Traumatic Sexualization/Eroticization		
Betrayal and Loss		
Stigmatization		
Powerlessness		
Self Blaming		
Destructive Acting Out		
Loss of Body Integrity		
Developmental Dissociative		
Development of Attachment Disorder		

Overall Trauma:

Concerns	Strengths

VII. Conclusions:

VIII. Recommendations:

Index

DATE			